Health and Social Disparity

JAPANESE SOCIETY SERIES
General Editor: Yoshio Sugimoto

Lives of Young Koreans in Japan
Yasunori Fukuoka

Globalization and Social Change in Contemporary Japan
J.S. Eades, Tom Gill and Harumi Befu

Coming Out in Japan: The Story of Satoru and Ryuta
Satoru Ito and Ryuta Yanase

Japan and Its Others:
Globalization, Difference and the Critique of Modernity
John Clammer

Hegemony of Homogeneity:
An Anthropological Analysis of Nihonjinron
Harumi Befu

Foreign Migrants in Contemporary Japan
Hiroshi Komai

A Social History of Science and Technology in
Contemporary Japan, Volume 1
Shigeru Nakayama

Farewell to Nippon: Japanese Lifestyle Migrants in Australia
Machiko Sato

The Peripheral Centre:
Essays on Japanese History and Civilization
Johann P. Arnason

A Genealogy of 'Japanese' Self-images
Eiji Oguma

Class Structure in Contemporary Japan
Kenji Hashimoto

An Ecological View of History
Tadao Umesao

Nationalism and Gender
Chizuko Ueno

Native Anthropology: The Japanese Challenge
to Western Academic Hegemony
Takami Kuwayama

Youth Deviance in Japan: Class Reproduction of Non-Conformity
Robert Stuart Yoder

Japanese Companies: Theories and Realities
Masami Nomura and Yoshihiko Kamii

From Salvation to Spirituality:
Popular Religious Movements in Modern Japan
Susumu Shimazono

The 'Big Bang' in Japanese Higher Education:
The 2004 Reforms and the Dynamics of Change
J.S. Eades, Roger Goodman and Yumiko Hada

Japanese Politics: An Introduction
Takashi Inoguchi

A Social History of Science and Technology in
Contemporary Japan, Volume 2
Shigeru Nakayama

Gender and Japanese Management
Kimiko Kimoto

Philosophy of Agricultural Science: A Japanese Perspective
Osamu Soda

A Social History of Science and Technology in
Contemporary Japan, Volume 3
Shigeru Nakayama and Kunio Goto

Japan's Underclass: Day Laborers and the Homeless
Hideo Aoki

A Social History of Science and Technology
in Contemporary Japan, Volume 4
Shigeru Nakayama and Hitoshi Yoshioka

Scams and Sweeteners: A Sociology of Fraud
Masahiro Ogino

Toyota's Assembly Line: A View from the Factory Floor
Ryoji Ihara

Village Life in Modern Japan: An Environmental Perspective
Akira Furukawa

Social Welfare in Japan: Principles and Applications
Kojun Furukawa

Escape from Work: Freelancing Youth and the Challenge to Corporate Japan
Reiko Kosugi

Gender Gymnastics: Performing and Consuming Japan's Takarazuka Revue
Leonie R. Stickland

Poverty and Social Welfare in Japan
Masami Iwata and Akihiko Nishizawa

Japan's Whaling: The Politics of Culture in Historical Perspective
Hiroyuki Watanabe

Health and Social Disparity in Japan: Japan and Beyond
Norito Kawakami, Yasuki Kobayashi and Hideki Hashimoto

The Modern Family in Japan: Its Rise and Fall
Chizuko Ueno

Social Stratification and Inequality Series

Inequality amid Affluence: Social Stratification in Japan
Junsuke Hara and Kazuo Seiyama

Intentional Social Change: A Rational Choice Theory
Yoshimichi Sato

Constructing Civil Society in Japan:
Voices of Environmental Movements
Koichi Hasegawa

Deciphering Stratification and Inequality: Japan and Beyond
Yoshimichi Sato

Social Justice in Japan: Concepts, Theories and Paradigms
Ken-ichi Ohbuchi

Gender and Career in Japan
Atsuko Suzuki

Status and Stratification: Cultural Forms in East and Southeast Asia
Mutsuhiko Shima

Globalization, Minorities and Civil Society:
Perspectives from Asian and Western Cities
Koichi Hasegawa and Naoki Yoshihara

Advanced Social Research Series

A Sociology of Happiness
Kenji Kosaka

Frontiers of Social Research: Japan and Beyond
Akira Furukawa

A Quest for Alternative Sociology
Kenji Kosaka and Masahiro Ogino

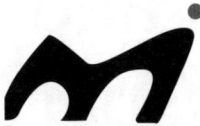

MODERNITY AND IDENTITY IN ASIA SERIES

Globalization, Culture and Inequality in Asia
Timothy S. Scrase, Todd Miles Joseph Holden and Scott Baum

Looking for Money:
Capitalism and Modernity in an Orang Asli Village
Alberto Gomes

Governance and Democracy in Asia
Takashi Inoguchi and Matthew Carlson

Health and Social Disparity

Japan and Beyond

edited by

Norito Kawakami
Yasuki Kobayashi

and

Hideki Hashimoto

Translated by
Kikuko Onoda

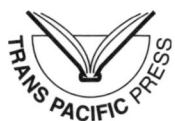

Trans Pacific Press
Melbourne

First published in Japanese in 2006 by the University of Tokyo Press as *Shakai kakusa to kenkō: Shakai ekigaku kara no apurōchi*.

First published in 2009 by
Trans Pacific Press, PO Box 164, Balwyn North, Victoria 3104, Australia
Telephone: +61 (0)3 9859 1112   Fax: +61 (0)3 9859 4110
Email: tpp.mail@gmail.com
Web: http://www.transpacificpress.com

Copyright © Trans Pacific Press 2009

Designed and set by digital environs, Melbourne, Australia. www.digitalenvirons.com

Printed by BPA Print Group, Burwood, Victoria, Australia

Distributors

Australia and New Zealand
UNIREPS
University of New South Wales
Sydney, NSW 2052
Australia
Telephone: +61(0)2-9664-0999
Fax: +61(0)2-9664-5420
Email: info.press@unsw.edu.au
Web: http://www.unireps.com.au

USA and Canada
International Specialized Book Services (ISBS)
920 NE 58th Avenue, Suite 300
Portland, Oregon 97213-3786
USA
Telephone: (800) 944-6190
Fax: (503) 280-8832
Email: orders@isbs.com
Web: http://www.isbs.com

Asia and the Pacific
Kinokuniya Company Ltd.

Head office:
3-7-10 Shimomeguro
Meguro-ku
Tokyo 153-8504
Japan
Telephone: +81(0)3-6910-0531
Fax: +81(0)3-6420-1362
Email: bkimp@kinokuniya.co.jp
Web: www.kinokuniya.co.jp

Asia-Pacific office:
Kinokuniya Book Stores of Singapore Pte., Ltd.
391B Orchard Road #13-06/07/08
Ngee Ann City Tower B
Singapore 238874
Telephone: +65 6276 5558
Fax: +65 6276 5570
Email: SSO@kinokuniya.co.jp

All rights reserved. No production of any part of this book may take place without the written permission of Trans Pacific Press.

ISSN   1443–9670 (Japanese Society Series)
ISBN   978–1–876843–52–6 (Hardcover)
ISBN   978–1–876843–58–8 (Paperback)

Cover illustration: Japanese sushi, globally believed to be healthy food.

Contents

Contributors	xiii
Acknowledgements	xiv
1 Social Epidemiology: Its Origins and Prospects	1
Part I: Economic and Social Programs, and Health	25
2 Poverty and Health	27
3 Income Distribution and Health	40
4 Access to Health Care and Health	66
5 Health and Occupational Class	90
Part II: Culture, Education, Social Relationships and Health	117
6 Education Inequality and Health	119
7 Gender and Health	144
8 Culture and Health	164
9 Social Relationships and Health	182
Part III: Research Methods and Ethics	209
10 Multilevel Analysis of Socioeconomic Factors	211
11 Social Epidemiology and Individuals, Society and Ethics	240
Appendix	259
Index	263

Figures

1.1:	Viewpoints of social epidemiology	2
1.2:	Social determinants of health status	11
2.1:	Vicious circle of poverty and disease	28
2.2:	Life expectancy and income per capita for selected countries and periods	34
3.1:	The relationship between income and life expectancy	41
3.2:	The relationship between all-cause, age-adjusted mortality rates and prefectural income distribution (Gini index) in 1995	44
3.3:	A hypothetical relationship between health status (risk) and income	47
4.1:	Conditions for having health care access	67
4.2:	Geographical accessibility to primary care	68
4.3:	Identified physician shortage areas in Illinois, USA	69
4.4:	Distribution of the variable percentage (%) of GPs achieving 80% targets in cervical screening for deprived and affluent areas	72
4.5:	Cervical cancer incidence and mortality rates	73
4.6:	The Lorenz curve and the Gini index	75
4.7:	Expenditure and illness shares, Netherlands 1981–1982	76
4.8:	Illness and expenditure concentration curves, Netherlands 1981–1982	77
5.1	SMRs, by social class (based on occupation), males, England and Wales, 1970–72, 1979–80, 82–83, and 1991–93	92
5.2:	Job demand–control model	93
5.3:	Effort–reward imbalance model	94
6.1:	Roles of health literacy in health promotion	122
6.2:	Schematic diagram of a model of associations between health literacy and health outcomes	132
7.1:	Three paradigms of biological and social sex, and health	150
7.2:	Prevalence of insomnia	152
7.3:	Prevalence of difficulty initiating sleep	153
7.4:	Prevalence of difficulty maintaining sleep	154
7.5:	Prevalence of hypnotic medication use	155

Figures

7.6:	Prevalence of poor sleep quality (among the general population)	157
7.7:	Prevalence of poor sleep quality (among workers)	158
7.8:	Concept of health and aging	161
8.1:	Hierarchical understanding of culture	167
8.2:	Positions of selected countries plotted on value dimensions	170
9.1:	Hierarchical structure of the determinants of health	183
9.2:	Marital status, marital satisfaction and depression ($\geq$ 10 points in GDS; results based on a general linear model adjusted for age)	188
9.3:	Social networks and mortality	191
9.4:	Age-adjusted mortality and lack of interpersonal trust	197
9.5:	Social capital and 'inappropriate care' (by school districts)	199
10.1:	Hierarchical data (of schools as an example)	213
10.2:	Types of contextual effect	215
10.3:	Association between age and blood pressure level – Example 1 (total number)	217
10.4-1:	Association between age and blood pressure level – Example 2 (by sex)	218
10.4-2:	Association between age and blood pressure level – Example 2 (by area)	219
10.5-1:	Association between age and blood pressure level – Example 3 (by sex)	220
10.5-2:	Association between age and blood pressure level – Example 3 (by area)	221
10.6:	Age-adjusted mortality rates by area- and individual-level variables (25-64 year-olds)	234
10.7:	Age-adjusted mortality rates by area- and individual-level variables (over 64 year-olds)	235

Tables

1.1:	Mortality rates by social classes in London in 1948	5
2.1:	An international comparison between an economic index and health indices (2002)	29
2.2:	Proportion of people living on less than one dollar a day (%)	30
2.3:	Mortality rates by gender and social class in the Black Report (15–64 years of age)	32
2.4:	Infant deaths by parental occupation in Kishiwada City (cumulative data from 1913 to 1935)	33
2.5:	Factors influencing health involving an individual and a nation, and their surrounding environments	36
3.1:	Prefectural income distribution, income levels and age-adjusted mortality rates	45
3.2-1:	A list of studies based on multilevel analysis using US and Japanese data (cross-sectional studies)	50
3.2-2:	A list of studies based on multilevel analysis using US data (longitudinal studies)	52
3.3:	An analysis of data from a 1995 Comprehensive Survey of Living Conditions of the People on Health and Welfare (N = 80899) (modified from Shibuya, et al. 2002)	56
4.1:	Results of logistic regression analysis of the probability that the consumption of prescription drugs would be reduced if the user charge (co-payment) increased	80
4.2:	Annual use of medical services per capita by plan (standard errors in parentheses)[a]	82
4.3:	Rates of adult medical-surgical hospitalisations by insurance plans[a]	85
4.4:	Factors associated with anti-HIV combination therapy (logistic regression analysis)	87
5.1:	Comparison of stress levels between occupationa classes based on demand–control model (JMS cohort study; baseline, 1992/1995)	97
5.2:	Relation between occupational classes and plasma-fibrinogen levels – results of multivariate linear regression analysis (JMS cohort study, 1992/1995)	98

5.3:	Relation between strain[a] and plasma fibrinogen by occupational class – results of multivariate linear regression analysis [b] (JMS cohort study, 1992/1995)	99
5.4:	Relationships between occupational classes and effort–reward stress indicators: age-adjusted odds ratios (OR) and 95% confidence intervals (95% CI) in regular workers under 60 years of age	102
5.5:	Comparison of effort–reward stress indicators between regular and non-regular workers: age-adjusted odds ratios (OR) and 95% confidence intervals (95% CI) in workers under 60 years of age	104
5.6:	Risk of depression calculated for different combinations of effort–reward imbalance and occupational class: odds ratios (OR), 95% confidence intervals (95% CI) and effects of interaction calculated by multivariate logistic analysis (in local public body employees, 2003/2004)	106
6.1:	Definitions of health literacy	120
6.2:	Previous studies on health literacy and social structure	124
6.3:	Previous studies on health literacy and health outcomes	128
6.4:	List of representative tools for health literacy assessment	135
7.1:	Differences in treatment by sex	149
8.1:	Associations between longevity measures, mode of death as a function of Chinese value dimensions and GNP/capita	172
8.2:	Frequency of use of acculturation measures in epidemiological studies on Asian immigrants	175
9.1:	Social network and social support	185
9.2:	Definitions of social capital appearing in research	195
10.1:	Types of fallacy in epidemiological studies	212
10.2:	Levels of subjects by types of analysis	214
10.3-1:	Age-adjusted mortality and mortality risk ratios by area-level and individual-level variables (25–64 year olds)	228
10.3-2:	Age-adjusted mortality and mortality risk ratios by area-level and individual-level variables (over 64 year olds)	230
10.4:	The effects of adjustments for area- and individual-level variables on the average relative deviation in area-level mortality	233

11.1: Recommendations for the role of epidemiology in the
       21st century   245
11.2: Ethical declaration on the conduct of epidemiological
       research   250
A.1: List of major events in and outside Japan relating to
       the establishment of the Japanese Ethical Guidelines
       for Epidemiological Research   259

Contributors

- Norito Kawakami, University of Tokyo, Japan
- Yasuki Kobayashi, University of Tokyo, Japan
- Hideki Hashimoto, University of Tokyo, Japan
- Satoshi Toyokawa, University of Tokyo, Japan
- Akizumi Tsutsumi, University of Occupational and Environmental Health, Japan
- Hiroki Sugimori, St. Marianna University School of Medicine, Japan
- Yuriko Doi, National Institute of Public Health, Japan
- Noboru Iwata, Hiroshima International University, Japan
- Katsunori Kondo, Nihon Fukushi University, Japan
- Nobuo Nishi, Radiation Effects Research Foundation, Japan
- Takeo Nakayama, Kyoto University, Japan

Acknowledgments

The publication of this book was supported by a Grant-in-Aid for Publication of Scientific Research Results from the Japan Society for the Promotion of Science. The editors are grateful to Ms Kikuko Onoda for her superb translation of our Japanese book. Thanks are also due to Mr Bill McCann for his excellent editorial support.

Norito Kawakami
Yasuki Kobayashi
Hideki Hashimoto

1 Social Epidemiology: Its Origins and Prospects

Norito Kawakami

What is social epidemiology?

Definition and characteristics

Many people would agree with the notion that society, economics and culture, including poverty, discrimination, social structure and employment, have an influence on people's health. Surprisingly, however, scientific demonstration and analysis of this notion has been lacking[1]. Social epidemiology is a new field of epidemiology which attempts to understand how social structure influences the distribution of health and disease, and to elucidate any mechanisms involved. Lisa Berkman and Ichirō Kawachi[2] define social epidemiology as the 'branch of epidemiology that studies the social distribution and social determinants of states of health'[1]. In the well-known tragedy, the sinking of the *Titanic*, the death rate was higher for passengers in steerage, located on the lower levels of the ship, than those in first-class cabins, located on the higher levels. Whether a passenger was in a first-class cabin or steerage depended on his or her socioeconomic status[3]. As seen from this example, a society's structure can generate the distribution of advantages and disadvantages, and this distribution, in turn, can generate the distribution of health and disease throughout the society. Social epidemiology is characterised by its attempt to understand the associations between social structure, individuals, and health and disease as forming multiple levels of reciprocal relationships (Figure 1.1)[4]. Social epidemiology has attracted attention as a new development in that it adds social points of view to the analysis of the relationships between socioeconomic factors and health – the relationships which have been focused on by conventional epidemiology mainly from individual and personal points of view.

Figure 1.1: Viewpoints of social epidemiology

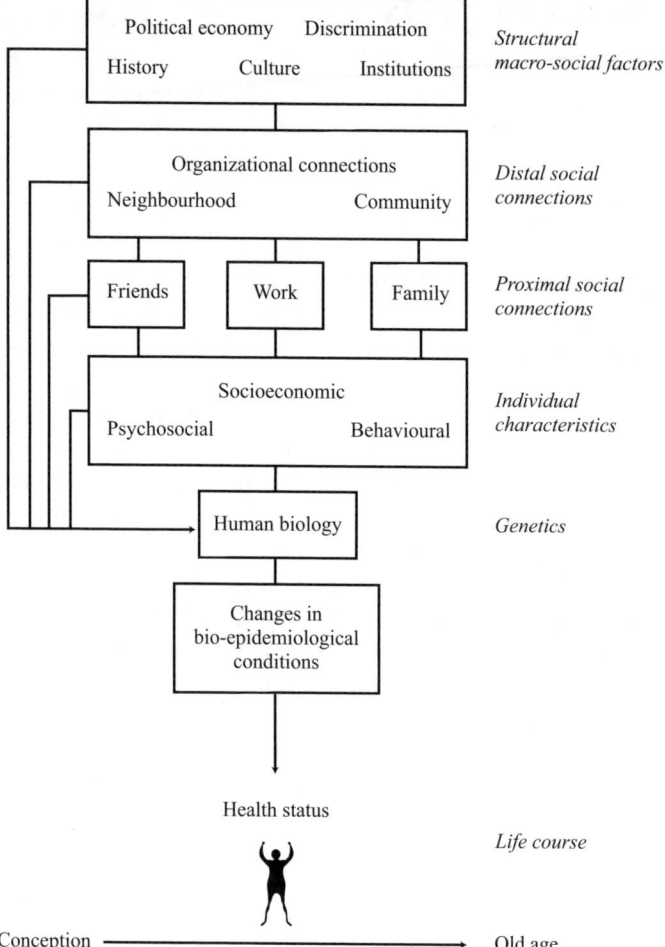

Note: Social factors generate health and disease through intervening variables. These processes accumulate and exert an influence on individuals throughout their lifetime.
Source: Figure 4 from Kaplan (2004 p.127)[4].

Social epidemiology as a field of epidemiology

Epidemiology is a science that attempts to find out the distribution, and its determinants, of health and disease in a given population and to solve health issues using the knowledge so obtained[5]. Social epidemiology is no exception to this definition. The history of epidemiology can be traced back to the ancient Greek era, when they discussed the relationship between climate and health. It would be fair to say, however, that modern epidemiological research started in the nineteenth century and the current system of epidemiology as a discipline was developed after the Second World War. Epidemiology has become a basic methodology for elucidating the relationships between people's environments or lifestyles and their health and for providing evidence-based medical services.

The main objective of epidemiology is to reveal a causal relationship between a certain factor and disease (or health). To this end, epidemiologists have refined indices of frequency and study designs. Epidemiological study results are particularly susceptible to potential bias in the sampling of subjects and the collection of information, and to the involvement of potential confounding factors, such as gender and age. Epidemiology attempts to exclude these biases as much as possible and to estimate causal relationships accurately.

Today's epidemiology has specialised into various fields, depending on the factors in question to which subjects are exposed, and on the diseases being examined. Fields of epidemiology based on exposure factors include environmental health and nutritional epidemiology. Those based on types of disease and health status include infectious disease epidemiology, cancer epidemiology and cardiovascular epidemiology. Social epidemiology fits into the former group, that is, a field which focuses on specific factors to which subjects are exposed[2].

Because of its name, social epidemiology is often misunderstood as a field which discusses the relationship between epidemiology and society or is interested in exerting an influence on society. Like many other fields of epidemiology, social epidemiology is very much interested in ploughing its findings back into communities. However, this does not differentiate it from other fields of epidemiology. What makes social epidemiology special is that it is interested in the influence of social structure on the health of individuals and populations, and attempts to elucidate the mechanisms of such influence within a multilayered framework consisting of social structures, people's behaviour and their health or disease.

History of social epidemiology

Classical approaches to social structure and health

The notion that social conditions and social structure have an influence on people's health emerged noticeably in the beginning of the nineteenth century, when the waves of industrialisation and urbanisation caused by the Industrial Revolution spread rapidly[6]. In France, Louis-René Villermé investigated death rates in poor and wealthy classes and proposed improvement in education and labour conditions in order to narrow the socioeconomic disparity in death rates. In Germany, after his assignment to Upper Silesia (part of today's Poland), Rudolph Virchow submitted a report to the German government in which he concluded through analysis that social disadvantages associated with certain social classes had an influence on the distribution of typhus. In his report, Virchow demanded reform of the region's administrative system, promotion of education, improvement of the social systems, including the tax system, and other economic measures[7]. In Britain, Edwin Chadwick published the *Sanitary Report* in 1948, in which he pointed out that in urban districts, major disparities had arisen in mortality between different social classes (Table 1.1)[8]. Through analysis, Chadwick concluded that the vicious circle of health problems and poverty in the working class was caused by poor sanitary conditions and the spread of infectious diseases in urban districts. Emile Durkheim used the term 'anomie' to describe a condition where social norms have broken down or been dissolved, and associated this condition with the occurrence of suicide. Durkheim believed that a lack of stability of social order, caused by extremely rapid changes in the community, may result in a loss of the authority of social norms which, in turn, may cause people to lose their standards of behaviour, making it likely for the community to fall into anomie. Durkheim seems to have pointed out the possibility that social structure may have an influence on people's mental health. These studies which focused on social structure and health were fairly advanced by the standards of their time. They were, however, unsophisticated in terms of the theories and methodologies on which they were based.

Development of theories in social epidemiology

In times when the major causes of death were infectious diseases, single causal factor theories dominated and these believe that a

Table 1.1: Mortality rates by social classes in London in 1948

	Proportion of deaths from infectious diseases to all deaths in each class (%)	Mortality of infants under 1 year of age	Proportion of deaths of children under 10 years of age to all deaths in each class (%)	Average age of death in each class	Average age of death of those who died at over 21 years of age in each class
Gentlemen, professionals and their families	6.5	1 in 10	24.7	44	61
Merchants, shopkeepers and their families	20.5	1 in 6	52.4	23	50
Wage earners, craftsmen, physical labourers and their families	22.2	1 in 4	54.5	22	49

Source: Table 2-1 from Hanlon (1974 p.18)[8]. Printed with permission from Elsevier.

specific disease is caused by a single agent. This was through the influence of bacteriology, which had developed dramatically with Robert Koch's discoveries of the anthrax bacillus (1876), the tubercle bacillus (1882) and the cholera bacillus (1883). In these theories, detection of the pathogen in the patient's body is a necessary condition for recognising the causal relationship between the pathogen and the disease, and all 'causes' other than the pathogen are ignored. This approach, however, does not apply to diseases which occur through the influence of various factors such as heredity, lifestyle and environment. Also, the development of infectious diseases is influenced by factors which increase the patient's exposure to the pathogen or which compromise the host's resistance. Hence, these ideas have resulted in the development of a new way of thinking on causal relationships which takes multiple factors into account. In today's epidemiology, a concept known as the 'web of causation', which argues that a disease occurs when multiple factors have interacted enough for the disease to occur, has become the mainstream[9].

Further, along with these multiple-factor models to explain disease, some epidemiologists began to consider it necessary to understand the influence of social structure on disease[2]. For instance, Graham Scambler emphasised that if smoking, poor nutrition and particular sexual behaviour are risk factors for diseases, they tend to concentrate in specific social classes. Scambler considered it necessary to understand why belonging to certain social classes may cause people to engage in risky behaviour and proposed to create a new area of epidemiology by uniting sociology and medical science.

In several fields of epidemiology, there gradually began to appear studies that focused on the relationships between social structure and diseases. One of them was psychiatric epidemiology, which is the epidemiology of mental disorders. Studies were accumulated on the links between socioeconomic class and the occurrence of mental disorders, from both of the following viewpoints: the possibility that people belonging to lower social classes may be more likely to develop mental disorders (social causation); and the possibility that people may shift to lower social classes because of their mental disorders; that is, genetic or family factors which make people more susceptible to mental disorders may cause them to shift to lower social classes (social selection). There was also an accumulation of epidemiological studies which discussed the relationships between physical diseases, on the one hand, and social class, status inconsistency, rapid social changes, cultural transformation and immigration, or social support and family ties, on the other. Based on the results of these studies, Mervyn and Ezra Susser, for instance, proposed the necessity of multilevel eco-epidemiology beyond the framework of conventional epidemiology which focused exclusively on personal factors[10].

Establishing stress science

The establishment of social epidemiology requires a biological explanation of how social structure exerts an influence on the health and diseases of human beings. Social structure could increase the exposure of people to risk factors or make people more likely to develop and maintain unhealthy behaviour. However, why do health problems become more likely to happen in situations where a rapid change, such as a social change, is occurring? Hans Selye discovered that the human body, in response to various outside demands, develops certain common (non-specific) responses, including hypertrophy of the adrenal cortex, atrophy of the thymus and lymph nodes, and gastric and duodenal ulcers. Selye named these responses 'stress'. Walter Cannon found in animal experiments that because of adrenaline released from the adrenal cortex, fear and other emotional responses result in physical changes, including increased cardiac rate, higher blood pressure and reduced gastrointestinal motility. The establishment of stress science, which links socio-psychological conditions and biological changes in the body that lead to disease, provided a theoretical foundation for social epidemiology.

Progress in strategies for public health and preventive medicine

In 1992, Geoffrey Rose published a booklet titled *The Strategy of Preventive Medicine*[11]. In this, Rose theoretically showed that risk factors for diseases are not distributed unevenly to create a group of high-risk people but that most of these risk factors, for example, blood pressure, are distributed continuously in a population; also that only a minor change in the average of a risk factor index may result in a significant change in the health status of a population or the occurrence of disease. Today, considering a population as a whole (the 'population strategy or approach') has come to be regarded as an important methodology in preventive medicine and public health, as is the idea of considering high-risk people (the 'high-risk approach').

In adopting a population approach, it is necessary to understand why there are differences in the distribution of risk factors between one population and another and to consider measures for addressing the differences. Elucidation of this problem requires viewpoints that are distinctly different from those required for clarifying the links between personal risk factors and disease occurrences.

In response to major changes in the nature of diseases over time, from infectious and chronic diseases to lifestyle-related diseases, the WHO advocated a strategy called 'health promotion' in its 1986 Ottawa Declaration. Health promotion is a strategy aimed at helping people to control and improve their own health. In particular, this strategy focuses not only on individuals' awareness and efforts, but also on the influence of various surrounding circumstances on people's health behaviour and health, including for example, their socioeconomic environment. In addition to health education approaches for improving individuals' lifestyles, it is essential to adopt approaches that work actively on the environment surrounding individuals, such as the creation of public health policies and/or a health-supporting environment. The WHO's concept of health promotion has been incorporated into the Japanese government's campaign for people's health in the 21st Century (Healthy Japan 21). This concept agrees with the view of social epidemiologists that social structure influences people's health. It is fair to say that the viewpoint of social epidemiology is essential in the promotion of population strategies.

Increase in public concern about socioeconomic differences

From the point in the nineteenth century when the Industrial Revolution was just over, developed countries at least, have progressively experienced significant improvements in sanitary conditions, progress in medical technology and increases in average longevity. As a matter of fact, however, the differences among social classes in health status, and disease and death rates have not necessarily been narrowed. Rather, there have been many reports showing increases in these differences. For instance, the differences in health status (including mortality from ischemic heart disease or IHD) among London civil servants in different occupations were virtually the same for the 1960s and the 1980s[12]. Between 1987 and 1994, smoking rates among US workers decreased in higher-status job categories, such as administrative or specialist positions, but remained at the same level for blue-collar workers. In addition, the differences in death rates among countries have been widening[13]. The WHO has shown strong concern over these continuing or widening socioeconomic differences in health status. European countries have a strong awareness of the socioeconomic differences as social issues, and many countries, including Britain and Sweden, have developed countermeasures against socioeconomic differences in health status. On the other hand, the USA has low awareness concerning the issue of these socioeconomic differences[14]. There have been various explanations for this. European countries have less movement of people between different income classes, and thus have more stable classes. Under these circumstances, these countries tend to regard widening of the income gaps as a problem. On the other hand, the USA has more movement of people between different income classes, which means these people have more opportunities to change their living conditions even though they may initially be poor. This has resulted in US citizens' low awareness of the issue[15]. Japan has long been said to be an 'equal' society, but in recent years it too has seen more and more inequality in income levels[16]. It has also been shown that more and more Japanese children have taken over their parents' occupations, which has resulted in ongoing loss of equal opportunity[17]. It seems that Japan, whose income classes are becoming more and more fixed like those of European countries, is another country where the necessity for social epidemiology is increasing.

Important concepts in social epidemiology

In these historical circumstances, the framework of social epidemiology, which focuses on the influence of social structure on people's health, had been formed by the 1980s. To help understand current social epidemiology, I will now present its important characteristic concepts.

Viewpoints integrating physical, psychological and social aspects

Social epidemiology emphasises viewpoints that integrate physical, psychological and social aspects (the biopsychosocial paradigm). Contemporary medicine focuses mostly on biological mechanisms, however, and it is essential to add psychosocial viewpoints to biological ones in order to understand the pathways through which social structure influences people's health. As already mentioned, it has been found, as a result of the development of stress science started by Selye's and Cannon's studies, that psychological stimuli (stressors), such as life events and difficulties in daily lives, have an influence on cardiac rate, blood pressure, blood-sugar level, immunological competence and other physical functions, through adrenaline and noradrenaline release which, in turn, occurs through the hypothalamus-pituitary-adrenal axis and sympathetic activations, respectively. It has also been found, as a result of accumulated studies in behavioural science, behavioural psychology and social psychology, that learning and social codes exert an influence on human behaviour. Based on these findings, it is believed that social structure creates social, work and material environments characteristic of each social structure, and that these environments have an influence on people's mental states and behaviour which, in turn, cause changes in the human body directly or through neuro-endocrine pathways (Figure 1.2). Social epidemiology attempts to understand the influence of social structure on people's health based on this model.

Social epidemiology also focuses on the viewpoint of a 'life-course' – the viewpoint that social structure's influence on a person's early life and cumulative influence on his or her entire lifetime are determinants of the person's health status. In the critical stages of human life, including foetal and childhood stages, a person's socioeconomic status exerts an influence on their exposure to malnutrition and infectious diseases. If an individual's exposure to disadvantageous social conditions lasts for a long time, the cumulative influence of the exposure will increase his or her risk of developing chronic disease.

Population strategy

As mentioned above, a population strategy is deeply related to social epidemiology. Let us assume that we are considering taking preventive action for residents in a community or workers in a particular workplace. The first idea that would come to mind is a high-risk strategy, in which people who are at high risk of contracting a certain disease are selected and receive the preventive action. However, let us take cerebrovascular disease as an example. It has a linear relationship with blood pressure as a risk factor. This means that people with high blood pressure are not the only ones who are at high risk of contracting cerebrovascular disease. As people without high blood pressure far outnumber those with high blood pressure, the majority of people who actually develop cerebrovascular disease do not have high blood pressure. In contrast, a population

Figure 1.2: Social determinants of health status

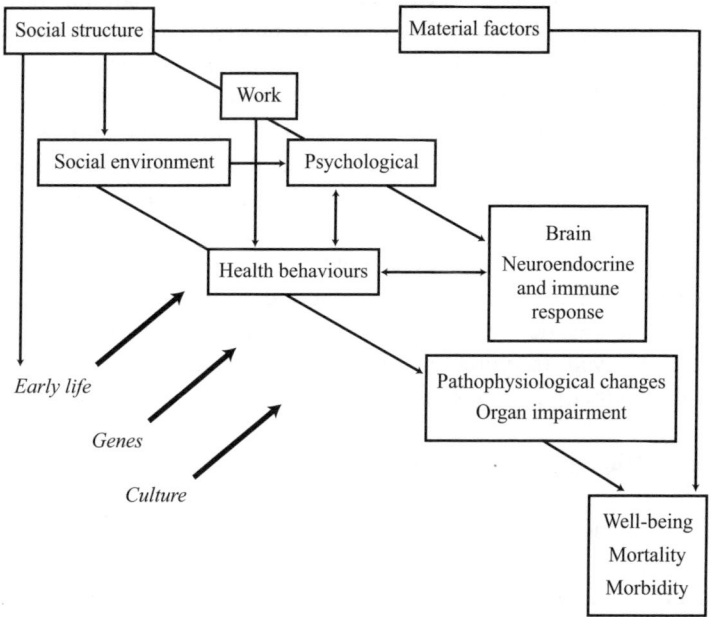

Note: Social structure exerts an influence on people's health and death through their material environment and mental/psychological, physiological and health behaviour.
Source: Marmot (1999)[20].

strategy attempts to prevent diseases by reducing the distribution of risk factors in the entire population. For instance, if a non-smoking campaign or a campaign for the separation of smokers from non-smokers directed towards the entire community results in a decreased rate of smoking, the health level of the population will improve. If the population is large, even a small decrease in the average of a risk factor index will produce significant preventive effects. Social epidemiological viewpoints and research results are useful in elucidating the cause of differences in the distribution of risk factors between different populations and in exploring measures to change the distribution. Social epidemiology is one of the methodologies supporting a population strategy.

Multilevel analysis and contextual variables

Multilevel analysis is one of the analytical methods often used in social epidemiology. Multilevel analysis uses information on exposures at both population and individual levels, and information on diseases at an individual level. For instance, a study has been conducted on the potential influence of living in low-income districts on health parameters, after adjustment for personal income. Exposure to the factors used in this study occurs at both levels: living in low-income districts is a factor, exposure to which occurs at the population level, whereas personal income is a factor at the individual level. In particular, factors at the population level often mean more than just the average of personal factors, and these factors are known as 'contextual variables'. Social epidemiology is interested in these variables which describe social structure or characteristics of the population associated with the social structure, and analyses, at multiple levels, the potential influence of population- and individual-level factors on people's health and disease.

Application of theories in sociology and psychology

In social epidemiology, theories and models developed in sociology, economics and psychology are actively used in proposing hypotheses and interpreting results. This use of theories, established as a result of the accumulated studies in related academic fields, makes it possible to interpret the multilayered, complicated relationships between social structure and an individual's health status. However, social epidemiology by no means ignores biological interpretation. Although some have expressed concern over potential confusion from carelessly bringing in theories from unfamiliar neighbouring fields of study[18], it will be a long time before all social relationships can be described using biological concepts and terms. At present, it is difficult to continue research in social epidemiology without the help of theories developed in related social sciences.

Main research fields in social epidemiology

Social class and health

The relationships between social class and health or disease are one of the main research topics in social epidemiology, and a large number of studies have been conducted on these relationships. A person's social class is usually determined by his or her income, property, education, occupation and so on. Studies have generally and consistently found that, in both developed and developing countries, people belonging to groups from lower social classes have poorer health status and higher prevalence of diseases than those among higher social classes. The same tendency has been found in a study which classifies social classes by occupation[12]. However, a comparative study between Japanese and European workers has found a weaker relationship between occupational positions and health status in Japan than in Europe, suggesting a possibility that some cultural differences may exist[19].

Economic levels, economic disparities and health

It has been known for a long time that low economic levels and poverty are related to poor health status and the occurrence of disease. The relationship between economic levels and health status can be observed conspicuously in comparisons between different countries. According to a report by the World Bank, for instance, there is an obvious correlation between GNP per capita and average longevity, namely, an increase in GNP is associated with increased average longevity. This link is particularly notable in countries with low GNP[20]. It is fully understandable that poverty would limit access to minimum necessities for people's health, including food, clothing, housing and medical services, resulting in poorer health. In recent years, attention has been focused on the fact that not only has the health status of the poor worsened, but extensive relationships have been observed between income levels and health status throughout communities. Some of these connections might mean that even for 'non-poor' people without any difficulty in obtaining necessities, a well-balanced nutrition, comfortable housing, private cars and other indices of affluence (which may or may not be available depending on one's income level) may have extensive links with health status. It has also been pointed out that material affluence, as measured by these indices, might contribute to people's health through socio-psychological satisfaction.

Investigation into the influence of income distribution (or income disparities) on health or disease is a field of study opened up very actively by social epidemiology. For instance, a comparison between Japan and European countries has shown that the more income disparities were reduced, the more average longevity increased[21]. In a study which used the Robin Hood index to represent sizes of the income disparities between different US states, and which investigated the relationship between the index and age-adjusted mortality rates, states with larger income differences had higher mortality rates[22]. In a community with a wide gap between rich and poor, the health status of the entire community may deteriorate because the rich and the poor often have different interests from each other, which may result in, for instance, fewer investments in public education and human resources development[6]. Alternatively, economic disparities may give rise to conflicts among people and may cause deterioration of people's health through crime, violence and social unrest. In addition, income disparities may relatively increase people's psychological sense of insufficiency or dissatisfaction, which may constitute psychological stress that leads to deterioration of health. In contrast, studies conducted in countries other than the USA have not clearly shown any influence of regional income disparities on health status[23]. It is inferred that any influence of income disparities tends to emerge under certain social systems.

Childhood experience, life history and health

The relationships between poverty, social inequality and discrimination on the one hand, and children's health issues on the other, are apparent in any country. Examples of biological factors damaging children's health include malnutrition and infectious diseases. Mothers' malnutrition and infectious diseases affect foetal development. Health problems in childhood affect a person's health status in adulthood. For instance, childhood malnutrition increases the risk of diabetes in adulthood. In addition, adverse socio-psychological factors in childhood, such as parental divorce, separation from parents or foster-child experiences, increase the risk of depression in adulthood. It also seems that socioeconomic factors in families play a role in the emergence of these childhood and pre-childhood biological and/or socio-psychological risk factors for ill health. Investigating the relationships between socioeconomic factors and health issues in childhood and adulthood is another area of social epidemiology.

Social epidemiologists also believe that adverse socioeconomic factors and other social disadvantages exert a cumulative influence on individuals throughout their life history and affect their health. According to a longitudinal study of US men, their fathers' occupations, years of education, initial occupations, occupations during middle age and property during middle age were associated with premature death (death before average life expectancy)[24]. In particular, a father's occupation was associated with the subject's education; and a higher education was associated with professional and other higher initial occupations, and a higher level occupation was associated with better socioeconomic conditions, influencing mortality rates. A Scottish longitudinal study has shown that the higher the frequency of working in lower occupations (physical labour) at various times in life, the higher the mortality, suggesting that accumulated frequency of exposure to unfavourable social conditions throughout a lifetime exerts an influence on health status[25].

Social support, social capital and health

Social relationships, measured by the number of, and the frequency of contact with family members, relatives and friends are called 'social networks'. Qualitative aspects of these social relationships, assessed by the quality of reliable relationships, the types of available support and satisfaction with the support, are called 'social support'. A large number of previous studies have found that better social networks and greater availability of social support were associated with lower mortality rates, lower occurrences of IHD, cerebrovascular disease and infectious diseases, and lower frequencies of depressive symptoms and mental disorders[26].

On the other hand, 'social capital' is defined as the characteristics of a community's views (norms) on the level of mutual trust, mutual interests and mutual aid. Social capital, which includes mutual trust and other elements, is the fundamental structure on which the population's social activities are based. Social capital serves to support individuals and to promote community action. It is also characterised by its function to produce public benefits instead of private benefits. Using the results of public opinion polls conducted in thirty-six US states, Ichirō Kawachi and his colleagues calculated the proportions of residents who responded that 'most people would try to take advantage of you if they got the chance' and investigated a potential correlation between these proportions and the respective states' mortality rates by age[27]. The results showed that the higher the proportion of people who responded that others were attempting to exploit them, the higher the mortality rate by age. The authors suggest that these results show the potential influence of the social sense of trust on health status.

Occupation and health

Assuming occupational class is one index of social class, it has been reported that lower occupational classes are associated with poorer health status. In addition, occupational stress has attracted attention as a factor for explaining the differences in health status among different occupational classes[12]. Epidemiological research into occupational stress has produced an accumulation of results on the influence of occupational stress on various aspects of health, ranging from IHD to mental disorders, based on the 'job demands-control model' or the 'effort–reward imbalance model'[28]. The proportion of people with 'high strain', characterised by high demands and low job control, is low in managerial, professional and technical jobs, and high among manufacturing and assembly workers, and physical labourers. Countermeasures against occupational stress may prove to serve as ways of narrowing the disparities in health levels among different occupational classes.

In recent years, the globalisation of corporate activities and the intensifying international competition among companies have caused one company after another to make drastic changes in their business and employment policies. In Japan, a large number of companies have given up lifetime employment and introduced a merit or pay-per-performance system. There have also been reports from the USA pointing out the influence of 'Just-in-Time', 'Kaizen' and other Japanese-style manufacturing methods on people's health. It is likely that this influence of companies' business, employment and personnel management policies on workers' health will become a matter of concern in future social epidemiology.

Discrimination and health

Discrimination can arise from differences of gender, race, language, disability, sexual orientation, age, income and other factors; and discrimination may affect people's health by producing advantages and disadvantages in the community[29]. Those who are discriminated against are placed in poor socioeconomic conditions, are vulnerable to violence and their pride always hurt. It has been reported that gender discrimination not only increases psychological stress, but also aggravates high blood pressure. It has also been reported that discrimination based on race, lifestyle, occupation and education exerts an influence on psychological stress, depression, smoking, high blood pressure and heart disease. In the USA, people live in different areas depending on their race and income levels, and it has been shown that differences in people's living areas exert an influence on their mortality rates.

Culture and health

The Ni-Hon-San Study, which investigated Japanese immigrants in the USA, found that the occurrence of IHD was highest among Japanese immigrants living in California, followed by ethnic Japanese in Hawaii, and then Japanese in Japan[30]. However, these differences could not be fully explained by blood pressure or total serum cholesterol levels. From this it was inferred that other cultural or behavioural factors may have played a role in the observed differences in the occurrence of IHD. Michael Marmot and his collegues[31] found that of the Japanese immigrants in the USA, those who had acculturated to the USA had a higher occurrence of IHD than those who had maintained their Japanese culture. In general, however, previous studies into the influence of acculturation (which takes place as a result of exposure to the destination culture) on migrants' health status or health behaviour (such as smoking and alcohol consumption) have shown that it is a complicated relationship[32]. Further research is warranted to understand the health issues which may be caused by immigration and acculturation.

A study[33] which compared US and Japanese workers showed that among US workers, higher frequency of contact with supervisors was associated with a markedly decreased sense of control and reduced job satisfaction. Conversely, for Japanese workers, higher frequency of contact with supervisors was associated with increased job satisfaction, suggesting a great difference in workplace culture and potential health influence. This kind of study on the differences in social structure between different cultures and countries provides us with important clues in elucidating the mechanisms working between social structure and health.

Measurement in social epidemiology

How does social epidemiology measure indices of social structure? For instance, social class is usually measured by income, education and occupation. Other often-used indices include ownership of a house and private car. In 1975, August Hollingshead proposed a composite index of socioeconomic status, consisting of four factors: sex, education, marital status and occupation. This index has been used in a large number of studies. Childhood social class is often measured by parental social class. Methods of classifying society based on occupation include, among others, a method which uses salary level and occupational position, and another which uses average standards of education, training and techniques required for different occupations. Some indices of social class have been used to measure regional levels. Proportions of white-collar or well-educated residents and the average income are examples of social class indices for measuring regional levels.

Income is an important measurement index in social epidemiology. An oft-used index is income adjusted for family size, which is calculated by dividing the pre-tax income (reported by the subject) by the number of household members. Sometimes, households with less income than half of the median for the country or region are classified as being in poverty, and this has often been used as an index of a low-income class. Alternatively, the average income of the subject's place of residence has often been used as an index of income for the population. In contrast, income disparities can serve as indices on a population basis only, and various indices used in the field of economics have been applied to studies in social epidemiology[34]. These include: the Gini index and the Robin Hood index; also the ratio of the proportion of households whose income is in the lowest ten percentile to the proportion of households whose income is in the top ninety percentile; the proportion of people whose household income is below the fifty, sixty or seventy percentile level; also the Theil entropy index and the Atkinson index. The Gini index is defined as one half of the average value of the absolute differences between all possible pairs of incomes of members of the population after normalising incomes of the entire population. A Gini index of zero (0) represents perfect 'equality', which means everybody has the same income, while an index of one (1) represents maximum 'inequality', meaning all available income is obtained by a single person. It has been reported that these indices of income disparity correlate fairly well with each other[35].

In the context of social relationships, macro-level studies have regarded the following, among others, as indices of social network resources: frequency of contact with groups to which, and the number of persons to whom, the subject is socially related. Meso-level studies have assessed social networks, using for instance the following aspects of social networks as indices: the social relationship size (i.e. number of persons), its density (i.e. frequency of contact with other members), and its number of functions. Micro-level studies have focused on psychological aspects of social support, and have described social support using such indices as qualitative assessments of reliable relationships and types of support received or available, and satisfaction with them. Furthermore, many studies have divided social support into emotional, instrumental, informational and appraisal supports, and so on. Methods developed to assess these aspects of social relationships include interviews and self-administered questionnaires. On the other hand, social capital represents views (norms) of a community on the level of mutual trust, mutual interests and mutual aid, and is a variable at the population level[36]. Attempts have been made to measure the level of social capital in target areas based on the following: a population's average response patterns to questions about mutual trust, such as whether most people are reliable (mentioned above); observation of residents' reactions to a stranger who asks them to lend him or her a small amount of money; and observation of the reactions of passers-by when they notice money on the street.

Social epidemiology attempts to measure factors which are generally considered difficult to measure, such as discrimination and acculturation. Methods of measuring levels of discrimination include: 1) assessment based on direct reports from individuals; 2) assessment by measuring differences in access to necessities and services available between those who are discriminated against and others; and 3) assessment using separation of living quarters based on race, et cetera.[29]. For acculturation, measurements that have been devised include: language and fluency; ethnicity of relatives, spouse and friends; participation in cultural activities; belief in one's own culture; and Westernisation of lifestyles[32]. However, none of these measurement indices are 'gold standards', and developing these indices is a research topic within social epidemiology.

From social epidemiology to health and social policies

Social epidemiology is not characterised by its application to society. However, social epidemiology is deeply interested in ploughing its results back into communities.

Social epidemiology is often criticised as useless because it deals with gender, race and other unchangeable conditions[18]. This is, however, an incorrect view. Even if these conditions are unchangeable, it is possible to obtain clues to improve people's health by elucidating the pathways through which differences in gender and race lead to social advantages and disadvantages, and then in turn to health and disease. For instance, the US Task Force on Community Preventive Health Services has recommended three measures based on previous research results in social epidemiology[37]. One of them is programs for young children aged three to five years to support the development of their social skills and preparation for entry to school. These school preparation programs aim to help children born to families in low socioeconomic circumstances surmount their disadvantageous conditions by exerting an influence on the children's interests and motivation and in time, education and employment. A second measure is house rental assistance programs. The USA has a shortage of houses available to low-income households, and people's living quarters have increasingly been separated based on social class, income, race and ethnicity. By using rental assistance coupons for low-income households that are issued by local governments, these programs have the following aims: to increase the range of houses available for rent by low-income households; to alleviate the separation of living quarters and improve public security in each community; and to reduce the amount of violence. The third measure is to adapt medical systems to different cultures. These systems aim to facilitate residents' access to, and improve the quality of, medical services by increasing the opportunities for residents with different linguistic and cultural backgrounds (such as immigrants) to consult health professionals who understand their respective languages and cultures. These measures have been developed based on an understanding of the mechanisms by which social structures exert an influence on people's health.

In 2003, the WHO Regional Office of Europe (WHO/Europe) produced the booklet *Social Determinants of Health – The Solid Facts*[38]. In this, WHO/Europe lists the following as social determinants of health and recommends socio-epidemiological measures with respect to each of them: the social gradient, stress, early life, social exclusion, work, unemployment, social support, addiction, food and transport. The viewpoints of social epidemiology are about to be put to practical use in health policies all over the world.

Social epidemiology deals with the influences of social structures on people's health. As such, social epidemiology is deeply involved in the design and planning of social systems to develop measures against such influences. This requires more accountability, more coordination with stakeholders and more transparency in decision-making processes than when developing ordinary health programs. In Japan, it is hard to say if it is possible to always establish sufficient transparency and reasonable procedures in the decision-making process for selecting social policies. However, recent years have seen the application of policy-making methods, such as inviting public comment, public hearings for citizens, and stakeholder discussion meetings, all of which are intended to ensure fair decision-making processes for addressing environmental and other issues[39]. It seems that consideration of community decision-making processes will become increasingly important in order for social epidemiology research to benefit communities.

Conclusion

Social epidemiology focuses on social disparities in health and disease which have been widening despite past efforts to improve health levels in the world. It attempts to elucidate this phenomenon using multilayered analysis of the correlation between social structure and disease, and to propose new preventive strategies. In Japan, too, widening income disparities and the progressive stratification of society have increased the necessity to understand the relationship between social structure, on the one hand, and human behaviour and health and disease on the other, in order to develop countermeasures to these trends. Also in response to this situation, we have seen increasing numbers of researchers and practitioners in epidemiology, medicine and various related fields of science who are interested in social epidemiology. Research and practical use of social epidemiology is also essential for the creation of a social environment which supports people's healthy behaviour as in Japan's health promotion strategy, Healthy Japan 21. This is because social epidemiology has a point of view that analyses, on multiple levels, the relationship between personal behaviour and health or disease from the aspect of social environment. Social epidemiology research in Japan has just started. This book presents the achievements of social epidemiology in Japan to date and shows its future tasks.

Literature

1 Hashimoto, H. (1996), 'Shakai ekigaku (Social epidemiology)', in Hideyasu Aoyama, Norito Kawakami and Shigeki Kōda (eds.), *Kon'nichi no ekigaku* (Today's Epidemiology), Tokyo: Igaku-Shoin, pp. 318–327.
2 Berkman, L. F. and I. Kawachi (2000), 'A historical framework for social epidemiology', in L. F. Berkman and I. Kawachi (eds.), *Social Epidemiology*, New York: Oxford University Press, pp. 3–12.
3 Hall, W. (1986), 'Social class and survival on the S.S. Titanic', *Social Science and Medicine*, 22 (6), pp. 687–690.

4. Kaplan, G. A. (2004), 'What's wrong with social epidemiology, and how can we make it better?', *Epidemiologic Reviews*, 26, pp.124–135.
5. Last, J. M. (ed.) (1988), *Ekigaku Jiten* (A Dictionary of Epidemiology), translated by Japan Epidemiological Association (2000), Tokyo: Japan Public Health Association.
6. Honjo, K. (2004), 'Social epidemiology; definition, history and research examples', *Environmental Health and Preventive Medicine*, 9 (5), pp. 193–199.
7. Schechter, M. (2003), 'Rudolf Virchow: public health, and the built environment', *Journal of Urban Health*, 80 (4), pp. 523–524.
8. Hanlon, J. (1974), *Public Health*, St. Louis: C. V. Mosby Company, 18.
9. Rothman, K. J. and S. Greenland (1998), *Modern epidemiology*, Philadelphia: Lippincott Williams & Wilkins.
10. Susser, M. and E. Susser (1996), 'Choosing a future for epidemiology: II. From black box to Chinese boxes and eco–epidemiology', *American Journal of Public Health*, 86, pp. 674–677.
11. Rose, G. (1992), *The Strategy of Preventive Medicine*, Oxford: Oxford University Press.
12. Marmot, M. G., G. D. Smith, S. Stansfeld, C. Patel, F. North, J. Head, I. White, E. Brunner and A. Feeney (1991), 'Health inequalities among British civil servants; the Whitehall II study', *Lancet*, 377, pp.1387–1393.
13. Marmot, M. G. (2005), 'Social determinants of health inequalities', *Lancet*, 365 (9464), pp. 1099–1104.
14. Kawachi, I. and B. P. Kennedy (2002), *The health of nations: why inequality is harmful to your health*, translated by N. Nishi, T. Nakayama, S. Takao and Shakai Ekigaku Kenkyū Kai (Social Epidemiology Research Group) (2004), Tokyo: Nippon Hyoron Sha.
15. Ōtake, F. (2003), 'Jakunen sō gyakuten kanō na shakai ni (Toward society where younger generation can reverse their situations)', *Nihon Keizai Shimbun*, 22 August 2003.
16. Tachibanaki, T. (1998), *Nihon no keizai kakusa – shotoku to shisan kara kangaeru* (Economic disparities in Japan – consideration from income and assets aspects), Tokyo: Iwanami Shoten.
17. Satō, T. (2000), *Fubyōdō shakai Nihon – sayonara sō chūryū* (Unequal society, Japan – good-bye all-middle-class nation), Tokyo: Chūō Kōron Shinsha.
18. Zielhuis, G. A. and L. A. L. M. Kiemeney (2001), 'Social epidemiology? No way.', *International Journal of Epidemiology*, 30, pp. 43–44.
19. Martikainen, P., E. Lahelma, M. Marmot, M. Sekine, N. Nishi and S. Kagamimori (2004), 'A comparison of socioeconomic differences in physical functioning and perceived health among male and female employees in Britain, Finland and Japan', *Social Science & Medicine*, 59, pp. 1287–1295.
20. Marmot, M. and R. G. Wilkinson (eds.) (1999), *Social Determinants of Health*, London, Oxford University Press.
21. Wilkinson, R. G. (1992), 'Income distribution and life expectancy', *British Medical Journal*, 304, pp. 165–168.
22. Kennedy, B. P., I. Kawachi and D. Prothrow-Stith (1996), 'Income distribution and mortality; cross-sectional ecological study of the Robin Hood Index in the United States', *British Medical Journal*, 312, pp. 1004–1007.

23 Subramanian S. V. and I. Kawachi (2004), 'Income inequality and health: what have we learned so far?', *Epidemiologic Reviews*, 26, pp. 78–91.
24 Mare, R. D. (1997), 'Socioeconomic careers and differential mortality among older men in the United States', in J. Vallin, S. D'Souza and A. Palloni (eds.), *Measurement and analysis of mortality: new approaches*, Oxford: Clarendon Press, pp. 362–387.
25 Smith, G. D., C. L. Hart, D. Blane, C. Gillis and V. M. Hawthorne (1997), 'Lifetime socioeconomic position and mortality; prospective observational study', *British Medical Journal*, 314, pp. 547–552.
26 Berkman, L. F. and T. Glass (2000), 'Social integration, social networks, social support and health', in L. F. Berkman and I. Kawachi (eds.), *Social Epidemiology*, New York: Oxford University Press, pp. 137–173.
27 Kawachi, I., B. P. Kennedy, K. Lochner and D. Prothrow-Smith (1997), 'Social capital, income inequality, and mortality', *American Journal of Public Health*, 87, pp. 1491–1498.
28 Karasek, R. A. and T. Theorell (1990), *Healthy Work*, New York: Basic Books.
29 Krieger, N. (2000), 'Discrimination and health', in L. F. Berkman and I. Kawachi (eds.), *Social Epidemiology*, New York: Oxford University Press, pp. 36–75.
30 Marmot, M. G., S. L. Syme, A. Kagan, H. Katō, J. B. Cohen and J. Belsky (1975), 'Epidemiologic studies of coronary heart disease and stroke in Japanese men living in Japan, Hawaii and California; prevalence of coronary and hypertensive heart disease and associated risk factors', *American Journal of Epidemiology*, 102 (6), pp. 514–525.
31 Marmot, M. G. and S. L. Syme (1976), 'Acculturation and coronary heart disease in Japanese-Americans', *American Journal of Epidemiology*, 104 (3), pp. 225–247.
32 Salant, T. and D. S. Lauderdale (2003), 'Measuring culture; a critical review of acculturation and health in Asian immigrant populations', *Social Science & Medicine*, 57 (1), pp. 71–90.
33 Lincoln, J. R. and A. L. Kalleberg (1990), *Culture, control, and commitment; a study of work organization and work attitudes in the United States and Japan*, Cambridge: Cambridge University Press.
34 Kawachi, I. (2000), 'Income inequality and health', in L. F. Berkman and I. Kawachi (eds.), *Social Epidemiology*, New York: Oxford University Press, pp. 76–94.
35 Kawachi, I. and B. P. Kennedy (1997), 'The relationship of income inequality to mortality: does the choice of indicator matter?', *Social Science & Medicine*, 45 (7), pp. 1121–1127.
36 Kawachi, I. and L. F. Berkman (2000), 'Social cohesion, social capital, and health', in L. F. Berkman and I. Kawachi (eds.), *Social Epidemiology*, New York: Oxford University Press, pp. 174–190.
37 Task Force on Community Preventive Health Services (2003), 'Recommendations to promote healthy social environment', *American Journal of Preventive Medicine*, 24 (S3), pp. 21–24.
38 Wilkinson, R. G. and M. Marmot (eds.) (2003), *Social determinants of health: the solid facts*, WHO Regional Office of Europe.
39 Fujigaki, Y. (2003), *Senmon chi to Kōkyō sei* (Public ethics and a spirit of specialism), Tokyo: University of Tokyo Press.

Part I
Economic and Social Programs, and Health

2 Poverty and Health

Yasuki Kobayashi

Poverty and disease

The relationship between poverty and disease is an age-old topic. The coordination between anti-poverty programs and various disease prevention programs has been a major issue in social medicine, public health, and social policy in general. In fact, the British physician and economist, William Petty, stated in the seventeenth century that investment in health was fully justifiable in light of the large number of lives that would be saved. In addition, the German physician and statesman, Rudolf Virchow, reported in the mid-eighteenth century, after inspecting an outbreak of plague in eastern Prussia, that its most likely causes were poverty and a lack of democracy. However, the relationship between poverty and disease is not as simple as saying one causes the other. It is a unique relationship in that poverty and disease can each be a cause and a result of the other, and they can also form a vicious circle (Figure 2.1).

In developed countries today, various social policies and welfare programs have virtually eradicated extreme poverty. Still, at a global level, there is a remarkable association between a country's affluence (or poverty) and its level of health. Table 2.1 shows a selection of developed and developing countries with large populations. Kenya, India and China, each whose gross national product (GNP) per capita is less than US$1,000, have clearly poorer health indices, such as shorter average longevity and higher under-five mortality, than the developed countries whose GNP per capita is much higher than US$10,000 dollars[1]. In general, a country's affluence and level of health seem to be closely related to each other. Upon closer examination however, the figures for China, among the developing countries, and those for the USA, one of the developed countries, may not be exactly consistent with the general trend. In fact, many complicated factors are involved in the comparison of poverty and health at an international level. This issue will be discussed in the latter half of this chapter.

Figure 2.1: Vicious circle of poverty and disease

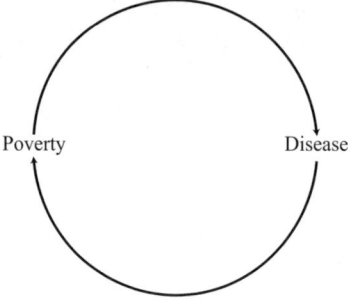

Definition and measurement of poverty

It is necessary to discuss the various definitions of 'poverty' before attempting an epidemiological analysis of its relationship to health; but arriving at a definition of poverty is not so self-evident.

There are two terms for defining and measuring poverty: 'absolute poverty' and 'relative poverty'. The former is based on the maintenance of life with a minimum of food and drink. The latter is based on a comparison with the living standards of the general public. Today, relative poverty is more popular as an approach to defining poverty, especially since the work of British sociologist, T. H. Marshall[2].

(Relative) poverty can be defined specifically by the following procedure, using the Engel coefficient (the proportion of food expenses in the total consumption expenditure): set a specific geographical area; calculate the amount of money required to purchase food for a minimum standard of living, taking nutritional considerations into account; and assume that the total expenditure of a household living on this amount of money is the minimum cost of living[2]. Thus, households living on a smaller budget than this minimum cost of living are defined as 'poor' and are considered to be targets for some kind of public assistance (e.g. welfare benefits). Even if this procedure is employed, however, a number of questions arise. For example, how should food required for a minimum standard of living be defined? What other expenditures besides food expenses should be allowed? In households owning land, savings and other assets, how should these be treated in the calculation? In addition, a means test, which scrutinises a subject's income, expenditure and assets, is not easy to accept for some people. Hence, even if one employs relative poverty as the definition of poverty, it is actually difficult to measure.

Table 2.1: *An international comparison between an economic index and health indices (2002)*

	Population (1 M)	GNP/capita (US$)	Health expenditure/GNP ratio	Under-5 mortality (in 1000 births)	Average life expectancy (years)
Kenya	31	360	8.3	114	49
India	1,025	450	4.9	94	61
China	1,292	780	5.3	37	71
Mexico	100	4,400	5.4	30	74
U.K.	60	22,640	7.3	7	78
Germany	82	25,350	10.6	5	78
U.S.	285	30,600	13	8	77
Japan	127	32,230	7.8	5	81

Source: World Health Organization (2004)[1].

Furthermore, different geographical areas and countries seem to have different definitions of poverty and different ways of measuring it. This is because prices of commodities, including food, are significantly different in different countries. Under these circumstances, international agencies have attempted various definitions of poverty. For a very specific and simple approach, the World Bank employs the following definition: 'living on less than US$1 a day'. In terms of the approaches to poverty described above, this would be an index of absolute poverty. The United Nations Millennium Development Goals (MDGs), which were agreed upon by the international community in 2000, aim at reducing the proportion of people living on less than one dollar a day in the world to fifty per cent of the 1990s level (one out of five people in the world) by 2015[3,4]. From Table 2.2, it can be seen that this goal will not be easy to achieve, and in fact, the situation deteriorated in some regions during the 1990s.

The Development Assistance Committee (DAC) of the Organization for Economic Cooperation and Development (OECD) defines poverty as a lack of the following five capabilities: political capability, social capability, economic capability, human capability and protective capability. The DAC then states that poverty does not arise solely from the lack of capabilities of individuals. It argues that different countries and regions have different structures causing poverty, where various factors are intricately linked and form a vicious circle that aggravates poverty.

Table 2.2: Proportion of people living on less than one dollar a day (%)

	1990	2001
Africa region	44.6	46.5
East Asia & Oceania region	29.6	15.6
Europe & Central Asia region	0.5	3.7
South Asia region	41.3	31.1
Latin America & Caribbean region	11.3	9.5
Middle East & North Africa region	2.3	2.4

Source: World Bank (2005)[3].

The Japan International Cooperation Agency (JICA), a Japanese government aid agency, employs a somewhat abstract definition of poverty: 'a condition in which people are deprived of their opportunities to demonstrate the potential capabilities required to lead a basic human life and are being left out of society and development processes.'

Hence, overall, various definitions of poverty have been described above; and while relative definitions have been widely used, it is clear that some African and Asian countries have a large number of people living in absolute poverty on less than US$1 a day.

Historical research on poverty and health

The Black Report

As typically seen with Edwin Chadwick, who played an active role in poverty relief measures and health administration during the mid-nineteenth century, Britain has for a long time paid attention to the relationship between poverty and disease, and this is reflected in its administrative programs. For instance, Chadwick started a disease registration project as part of relief measures for the poor, and established a foundation for statistical investigation of the relationship between disease and socio-environmental factors. This made the relationship between poverty and disease amongst workers in a capitalist society much clearer[5].

More recently, in 1980 the well-known Black Report was commissioned and later published by the British government (Ministry of Health and Social Security)[6]. This Report stated that in all age brackets, for both men and women, the mortality rates were higher in relatively lower socio-occupational classes. (Table 2.3 shows the mortality rates by gender in people between fifteen and sixty-four years of age). Four explanations have been proposed to interpret this phenomenon[6,7,8]. 1) The 'artefact explanation': this suggests that the investigation and statistical data are inaccurate and biased, resulting in an apparent association that does not actually exist. However, the effects of any inaccuracy and bias seem to have been substantially eliminated by subsequent verification using more accurate data. 2) The 'social selection explanation': this suggests that some people shift to lower socio-occupational classes due to ill health or disease, while some shift to higher classes due to good health. As a result, an association is seen between socio-occupational class and health status. Alternatively, an association may exist between people's levels of education (or intellect) and health status as a result of indirect social selection. People with higher education are more likely to have knowledge and understanding of healthy lifestyles and risk factors of diseases, more likely to try to maintain healthy lifestyles, and achieve socio-occupational success by making use of their education and/or intellectual capabilities. This results in the association between socio-occupational class and health status. 3) The 'behavioural and cultural explanation': this is related to the ideas described in (2) above and (4) below. It suggests that a person's specific pattern of behaviour (smoking, alcohol consumption, risky behaviour, etc.) is closely associated with the person's socio-occupational class and disease occurrence. 4) The 'materialist/structural explanation', which argues that being in lower social and income classes results in an inability to purchase goods and services necessary to maintain health which, in turn, results in higher disease prevalence and mortality rates. Clearly, these four hypotheses are related to the social epidemiological topic of this chapter.

Research on infant deaths in Japan

In Japan too, mainly during the 1930s, the researcher Dr. Hiroshi Maruyama actively investigated and analysed the relationship between parental occupational class and infant mortality rates, and became known for proposing the 'alpha index'. This index is calculated by dividing infant mortality (number of deaths in infants under the age of one year) by newborn mortality (number of deaths in infants under four weeks of age). It has the advantage of being able to be calculated from numbers of deaths only (and statistics

Table 2.3: *Mortality rates by gender and social class in the Black Report (15–64 years of age)*

Socio-occupational class	Males	Females	M/F ratio
I. Professional jobs	3.98	2.15	1.85
II. Intermediate jobs	5.54	2.85	1.94
III N. Managerial and engineering jobs	5.80	2.76	1.96
III M. Skilled jobs, manual labour	6.08	3.41	1.78
IV. Semi-skilled jobs	7.96	4.27	1.87
V. Non-skilled jobs	9.88	5.31	1.86
V/I ratio	2.50	2.50	N/A

Note: Per 1,000 population. England and Wales. 1971.
Source: Table 1 from Black, et al. (1982)[6].

of deaths are generally easier to research than births). The value of an alpha index becomes smaller as deaths due to infectious disease or other acquired causes decrease. Use of the alpha index makes it relatively easy to ascertain the health level of a target region.

Maruyama and his colleagues believed that infant mortality represents the health status of a community quite well. Based on this belief, they conducted a meticulous study in Kishiwada City in Osaka, Japan, where they transcribed death and stillbirth registrations and conducted interviews at maternity clinics and homes. The researchers analysed the status of infant mortality and its potential association with parental occupation[9]. They were unable to calculate the mortality rate because of an inability to investigate birth registrations. Nonetheless, they calculated the number of infant deaths per household by occupational classes (Table 2.4). Although these figures can provide only limited information (because precise numbers of births are unknown), they are invaluable data from that time. Maruyama and his colleagues also estimated the infant mortality rates for all Kishiwada City for the fifteen years, 1916 to 1930, and showed that they were approximately five times higher than the values for the nobility provided in another contemporaneous report. Dr. Maruyama certainly mentioned various issues concerning the definition of infant death and methods of surveying infant deaths in those days, and added that his data might not be very precise. Despite this, his study must have been pioneering work in social epidemiology in Japan.

Table 2.4: *Infant deaths by parental occupation in Kishiwada City (cumulative data from 1913 to 1935)*

	Infant deaths	Number of households	Infant deaths/ 100 households
Agriculture & fisheries	589	923	64
Manufacturing & mining	1,477	2,867	51
Commerce	1,450	2,732	53
Public service & freelance	570	912	63
Labour & traffic service	576	1,470	39
Unemployed	578	859	67
Household servants	–	239	–
Total	5,240	10,004	52

Source: Table 1-10, partially modified, from Maruyama (1976)[9].

World Development Report 1993

The *World Development Report* is published annually by the World Bank with a different theme each year. The 1993 Report is titled 'Investing in Health' and features a wide range of health issues in a wide range of countries, particularly developing ones. The issues include people's health levels, the organisation of health and medical systems, health and medical expenditures by households and governments, health and medical policies, and levels of public health[10]. The 1993 Report also proposes three approaches for governmental policies to improve health levels in developing countries: first, governments must promote an economic environment which will enable family budgets to improve the health of family members. Particularly important is investment in the primary school education of girls. Second, governments should give a higher priority to cost-effective health and medical programs. Third, governments must promote diversity and competition in both the sources and supply of health and medical services. For example, governments should invest predominantly in public health and basic medical services, and should consider contracting out other services to the private sector. These three approaches encountered some criticism as they were policies based on economic efficiency and market mechanisms. The Report represented, however, a landmark set of recommendations and demonstrated the World Bank's high level of concern over health and educational issues.

Figure 2.2: Life expectancy and income per capita for selected countries and periods

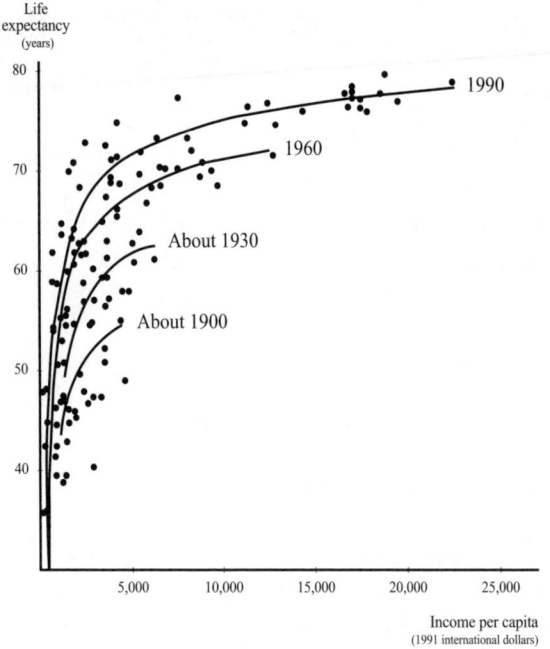

Note: International dollars are derived from national currencies, not by use of exchange rates but by assessment of purchasing power.
Source: Figure 1.9 from World Bank (1993)[10].

The 1993 Report illustrates the relationship between income per capita and average life expectancy in various countries and is evidence of a close association between the level of affluence and the level of health of a country. Figure 2.2 shows quite a strong correlation between average life expectancy and income per capita in these countries throughout the twentieth century. For this period, there was also a tendency that in countries whose income per capita was less than US$3,000, an increase in income was associated with a rapid increase in average life expectancy. Generally, therefore, it seems possible to improve the health status of a country if it can achieve a certain level of income. On the other hand, countries with the same level of income do not necessarily have the same health status; some have a good standard and others a poor standard. Thus, while it is clear that the health level of a country does not depend solely on its level of affluence, it would be fair to say that the *World*

Development Report 1993 shed new light on poverty and health issues at a global level.

Mechanisms by which poverty affects health

The mechanisms by which poverty and social deprivation cause deterioration of health levels and specific diseases are central issues in social epidemiology. For a description of various hypotheses on these mechanisms, please refer to Chapter 1. This section focuses mainly on poverty and health, the most direct mechanism involved, and is the basis for the title of this chapter.

As described above, poverty today is quite different between developed and developing countries. Poverty in developed countries is most often 'relative poverty' and can be clearly distinguished from 'absolute poverty' in developing countries. In fact, many developed countries have a welfare system which, if not perfect, allows most people to live on at least US$10 a day. If differences in commodity prices are taken into account, and even more so, if differences in housing and living environments are considered, poorer people in developed countries are in quite a different situation from those in absolute poverty, living on less than US$1 a day in developing countries. It is not difficult to imagine that failure to meet basic living requirements (such as provision of safe water, good nutrition, housing, environmental hygiene and public security), can lead to ill health among the poor in developing countries. The mechanism for this is explained to a considerable extent by two of the hypotheses mentioned above (in the section on the Black Report), namely, the 'materialist/structural explanation' and part of the 'behavioural and cultural explanation' (particularly the lack of primary education, etc)[8,11].

Table 2.5 shows factors influencing health, categorised into those involving an individual and his/her immediate environment, and those involving the nation and its surrounding environment. This is an easy way to understand these factors when considering measures to be taken. For an individual and their surrounding environment, health is significantly influenced not only by conventional epidemiology factors, such as individual characteristics and lifestyles, but also by social epidemiology factors, such as income, class and social capital. Important measures to be taken would include health education, anti-smoking promotions, and nutritional counselling, which can all be conducted on an individual level; and health projects, welfare activities, creation of support systems

Table 2.5: Factors influencing health involving an individual and a nation, and their surrounding environments

---

Factors involving an individual and their surrounding environment
    Individual variation (heredity, background), lifestyle, income, occupation, social class, social capital, etc.

Factors involving a nation and its surrounding environment
    Natural conditions (climate, topography, natural disasters, etc.)

    International conditions (war, international situation, foreign debt, etc.)

    Internal conditions (public order, employment, economic policy, food policy, educational system, cultural/social customs, class system, etc.)

    Health and medical conditions (living environment, public hygiene/health policy, access to medical services, healthcare system, etc.)

---

and construction of social networks, all of which can be managed at local or regional administrative levels. On the other hand, at the national level, it is no exaggeration to say that climate, war and national systems and policies, including public health policies, have a significant influence on the health of those in absolute poverty who cannot easily improve their surrounding environment. It is difficult to make a country rich immediately, but it would seem possible to raise the level of health of its people by political intervention at a national level in such areas as education and public health. It would be fair to say that this is exactly what was emphasised by Chadwick in Britain in the mid-nineteenth century, and by the 1993 *World Development Report*.

Recent studies

Many studies have been conducted on the influence of poverty (low income) on health since the Black Report. However, poverty is closely associated with factors such as age, gender, race, ethnicity, socio-occupational class and living environment, and it is difficult to isolate the influence of income.

Recently, multilevel analysis which pays attention to the hierarchical structure of data has been employed when handling individual-level variables (e.g. income, age, gender) and regional- or population-level variables at the same time. In addition, quite a few reports have suggested that income distribution (income disparity) within a population matters more than individual income levels. Research on this subject has been actively promoted (and is detailed in Chapter 3).

The analysis by Subramanian and colleagues of mortality rates in Massachusetts, USA, has shown that the association between poverty and mortality is particularly notable in the black population[12]. In Healy's comparative study of fourteen EU countries, there is an association between the percentage of people living in poverty and excess winter deaths, independent of income disparities[13]. A cohort study conducted by Osler and colleagues in Denmark has found that when households are divided into four categories based on individual income, lower all-cause mortality is associated with higher household income, with the ratio of the mortality rate for the highest-income households to that for the lowest-income households being 0.64 (95% confidence interval [CI], 0.57–0.73) and 0.68 (95% CI, 0.65–0.89) for men and women, respectively, with all other risk factors controlled[14]. Based on the results of a nationwide follow-up study in the USA, Fiscella and Franks have reported that the association between mortality rate and regional income disparity disappears when adjusted for household income[15].

In Japan, it is said that the largest income disparities are found among the elderly. At all the acute care hospitals in one particular prefecture, this author and colleagues surveyed patients who were admitted urgently because of strokes, and inquired after the patients' condition one year after their admission. A statistical association was found between the patients' return to home after discharge, and a lack of financial support from their families (basically, being able to live on a pension)[16]. This means that the economic conditions of the elderly themselves are associated with the place where they are taken care of, and this situation may influence the prognosis of their disease that will follow. In former epidemiological studies in Japan, many subjects gave no response to direct questions about their income. This caused a lot of researchers to ask the subjects about their economic conditions using indirect expressions, such as 'life circumstances'. Recently, however, large-scale social epidemiological surveys which involve the collection of accurate income information have started, based on the understanding that income disparities are widening in Japan. These surveys have reported an association between income and subjective health perception[17,18]. It is likely that these studies will be able to conduct a detailed analysis of the association between poverty (low income) and health in Japan, and will elucidate the mechanisms connecting these two states.

Literature

1 World Health Organization (2004), *The World Health Report 2004*, Geneva: WHO.
2 Konuma, T. (1980), *Hinkon – sono sokutei to seikatsu hogo* (Poverty – its measurement and livelihood protection), 2nd edition, Tokyo: University of Tokyo Press.
3 World Bank (2005), *Sekai kaihatsu hōkoku* 2005 (World Development Report 2005), Tokyo: Springer-Verlag.
4 Ministry of Foreign Affairs (2005), Millennium Development Goals, website of Official Development Assistance of the Ministry of Foreign Affairs (*http://www.mofa.go.jp/mofaj/gaiko/oda/index.html*).
5 Tatara, K. (1999), *Kōshū eisei no shisō – rekishi kara no kyōkun* (Ideas of public health – lessons from history), Tokyo: Igaku Shoin.
6 Black, D., J. N. Morris, C. Smith and P. Townsend (1982), *Inequalities in health; the Black Report,* Harmondsworth: Penguin.
7 Macintyre, S. (1997), 'The Black Report and beyond: what are the issues?', *t*, 44, pp. 723–745.
8 Shaw, M., D. Dorling and G. D. Smith (1999), 'Poverty, social exclusion, and minorities', in M. Marmot and R. G. Wilkinson (eds.), *Social determinants of health*, Oxford: Oxford University Press, pp. 211–239.
9 Maruyama, H. (1976), *Shakai igaku kenkyū I: nyūji shibō* (Social medicine research I: infant deaths), Tokyo: Iryō Tosho Shuppan Sha.
10 World Bank (1993), *World Development Report 1993*, Oxford: Oxford University Press.
11 Lynch, J. W., G. D. Smith, G. A. Kaplan and J. S. House. (2000), 'Income inequality and mortality: importance to health of individual income, psychosocial environment, or material conditions', *British Medical Journal,* 320, pp. 1200–1204.
12 Subramanian, S. V., J. T. Chen, D. H. Rehkopf, P. D. Waterman and N. Krieger. (2005), 'Racial disparities in context; a multilevel analysis of neighbourhood variations in poverty and excess mortality among black populations in Massachusetts', *American Journal of Public Health*, 95, pp. 260–265.
13 Healy, J. D. (2003), 'Excess winter mortality in Europe: a cross country analysis identifying key risk factors', *Journal of Epidemiology and Community Health,* 57, pp. 784–789.
14 Osler, M., E. Prescott, M. Gronbaek, U. Christensen, P. Due and G. Engholm. (2002), 'Income inequality, individual income, and mortality in Danish adults: analysis of pooled data from two cohort studies', *British Medical Journal*, 324, pp. 1–4.
15 Fiscella, K. and P. Franks (1997), 'Poverty or income inequality as predictor of mortality: longitudinal cohort study', *British Medical Journal,* 314, pp. 1724–1727.
16 Tamiya, N., Y. Kobayashi, S. Murakami, J. Sasaki, K. Yoshizawa, J. Otaki and K. Kano (2001), 'Factors related to home discharge of cerebrovascular disease patients: 1-year follow-up interview survey of caregivers of hospitalized patients in 53 acute care hospitals in Japan', *Archives of Gerontology and Geriatrics*, 33, pp. 109–121.

17 Yoshii, K., K. Kondō, H. Hirai, R. Matsuda and Y. Saito (2005), 'Kōreisha no shinshin kenkō no shakai keizai kakusa to chiiki kakusa no jittai (True state of socio-economic disparities and regional disparities in mental and physical health of the elderly)', *Kōshū eisei* (Journal of Public Health Practice), 69 (2), pp. 145–148.
18 Yamazaki, S., S. Fukuhara and Y. Suzukamo (2005), 'Household income is strongly associated with health-related quality of life among Japanese men but not women', *Public Health*, 119, pp. 561–567.

3 Income Distribution and Health
Hideki Hashimoto

Introduction: from income level to income distribution

As outlined by Yasuki Kobayashi in Chapter 2, it seems clear that there is a close association between economic/income level and health, and that raising people's living standards is an effective way of improving their levels of health. In developed countries where people's living standards have reached a somewhat satisfactory level then, does this kind of poverty-health issue no longer exist? A debate over this issue was kindled by Richard Wilkinson's paper, 'Income distribution and life expectancy', published in 1992[1] (Figure 3.1).

The vertical axis of the figure shows an increase in life expectancy over the period shown. The horizontal axis shows the ratio of the total income earned by people in the lower sixty percentile (when ranked by household income) to the total income earned by all households in the country. Specifically, the lower the ratio, the wider is the disparity between the lower-income class and the higher-income class. The figure shows that the wider this disparity in a country is, the smaller the increase tends to be in the life expectancy of the country. While it has commonly been found that absolute economic/income level has an influence on health, the above data suggests the possibility that in a given population, the disparity of income distribution, or relative income level, may also have an influence on people's health.

Since the collapse of the former Soviet Union and their introduction of a capitalist economy, Russia has achieved satisfactory economic development as assessed by macroscopic indices, including gross national product (GNP). However, its population's life expectancy has actually decreased. This is considered to have resulted, at least partially, from the increased disparities between rich and poor, caused by the rapid introduction of a free market economy[2]. Recently in Japan, too, the widening of income disparities and the class stratification of consumer behaviour have started attracting attention[3,4], after the collapse of the bubble economy.

Figure 3.1: The relationship between income and life expectancy

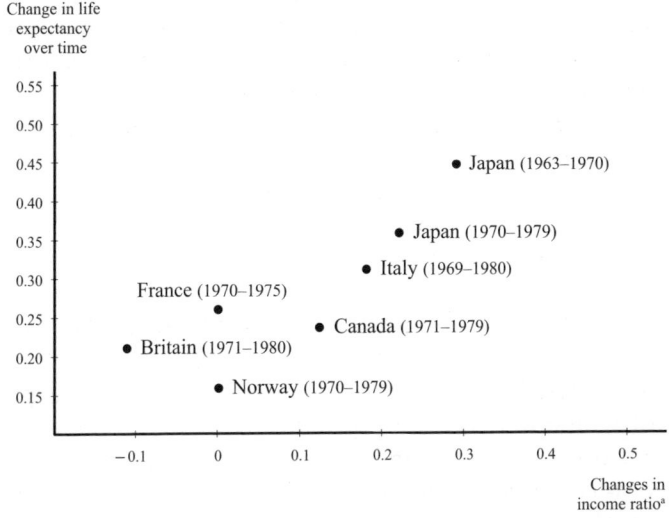

Note.

a: Changes in ratio of total income earned by people in the lower 60-percentile of the total population to total income earned by the total population (the higher the ratio, the smaller is the disparity).

Source: Wilkinson (1992)[1]. Figure modified with approval from BMJ Publishing Company Group.

The idea that disparities between the rich and poor affect people's health is intuitively very easy to understand. However, studies to demonstrate this are still struggling through unsettled theoretical and methodological debates. The preceding chapter discusses mainly the influence of absolute income level or absolute deprivation. In contrast, this chapter aims to discuss the influence of income distribution, or relative deprivation, based on research conducted in Japan and other countries, and other available empirical data.

First, the following section will discuss the macro-level relationship between local mortality rates and income disparity, based on data from Japanese and other national studies. As described below, most macro-level studies report an association between mortality rates and income disparity indices. In macro-level studies, however, it is impossible to eliminate the effects of confounding variables, such as personal income, and it is thus difficult to distinguish between the influence of absolute income level and that of relative income level (income distribution/disparity). Then a later section will summarise the results of studies conducted in Japan and elsewhere which use so-called multilevel data and take personal income and attributes into account. As we sort out the arguments around the question of whether health is affected by absolute personal income levels or local income disparities, a new question arises. Finally, a comparison will be made of three major hypotheses concerning the mechanisms by which income level affects people's health. This will be followed by a few comments on theoretical and methodological issues, and some implications for social epidemiological studies on income distribution and health in the future.

Empirical studies with macro-level (ecological) data

Wilkinson's study, mentioned in the preceding section, was exposed to criticism of the quality of its data and its analytical methods. The results of later re-examinations have denied any significant association between mortality rate and income level for comparative international data[5, 6]. As it is unreasonable to make a direct comparison between countries with different systems and political cultures, subsequent studies dealt with a potential association between income disparity and health indices within one country. Most published studies compared different states in the USA. Many of these studies have found a significant association between all-cause, age-adjusted mortality rates and income disparity[7-9]. However, few reports have been produced from other countries on these kinds of studies of macro-level data. An example of a study conducted by this author in Japan is described below. Figure 3.2 shows a graph of all-cause, age-adjusted mortality rates as a function of income disparity (Gini index) by prefecture[10].

A tendency can been seen in that the larger the income disparity in a prefecture, the higher the age-adjusted mortality rate. In fact, the Pearson correlation between these two variables is 0.21 ($p = 0.14$) [exclusion of the extreme observation from Okinawa Prefecture, where the mortality was extremely low in spite of having the highest Gini Index, would result in a considerable increase of the correlation to 0.42 ($p < 0.01$)]. Table 3.1 shows the results of analyses of the same data by gender and by age group (0–14, 15–59 and ≥60 years of age).

The table indicates the following results:
1. For both genders, a significant positive association was found between age-adjusted mortality rates for all age groups combined, and the prefectural Gini index. In other words, the

wider the disparity in a prefecture, the higher was its mortality rate.
2. However, observation by age group revealed that the above tendency (1) was clearly seen only in those 15–59 years of age.
3. If prefectural median income was included in the analysis, however, the positive association between the mortality rate and Gini index above disappeared. Instead, a negative association was actually found between mortality rate and prefectural median income in the 15–59 age group. In other words, the higher the income of a prefecture population, the lower was its mortality rate among the age group. This means that the relatively powerful negative association between the Gini index and prefectural median income (-0.51) results in a confounded association between the mortality rate and the Gini index.
4. For those at or above 60 years of age on the other hand, income disparity showed a positive association with mortality rate, even if the influence of prefectural median income was controlled. That is, the wider the prefectural income distribution disparity, the higher was its mortality rate. The relationship between prefectural median income and mortality rate in this age group was a positive one, the opposite of that for the 15–59 age group (namely, the higher the prefectural income, the higher was its mortality rate).

These tendencies remain even if the analysis is limited to the following specific causes of death: malignant neoplasm, ischemic heart disease and cerebrovascular disease. Thus, the following conclusions can be drawn with respect to the relationship between prefectural age-adjusted mortality rate and income level/distribution disparity in Japan in 1995:
1. The relationship between income disparity and mortality rate was strongly confounded by median income level.
2. After controlling for median income level, the positive relationship between income disparity and mortality rate lost statistical significance, except for the elderly strata.
3. The direction of correlation between median income level and mortality rate varied across different age groups: negative among the younger population and positive among the elderly.

In fact, none of the above findings holds true for previous US studies in which the influence of income disparity remained significant

Figure 3.2: The relationship between all-cause, age-adjusted mortality rates and prefectural income distribution (Gini index) in 1995

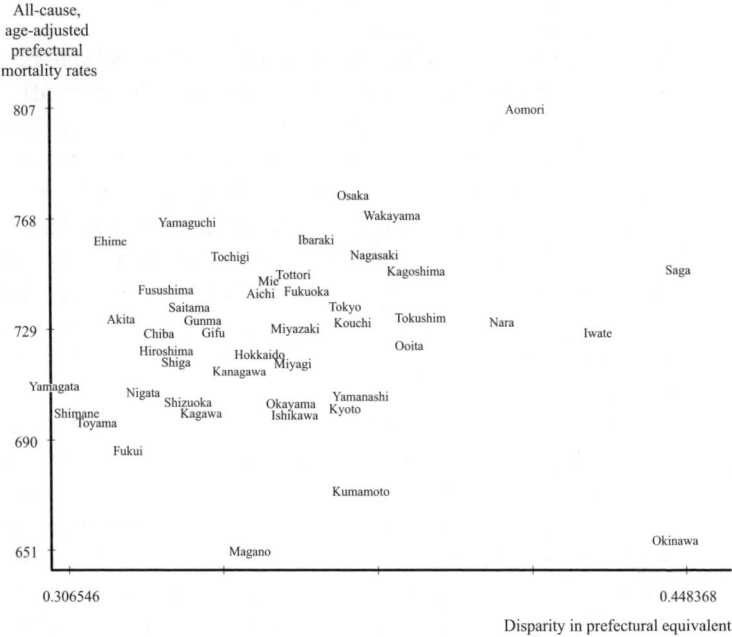

even after the state median income had been adjusted[7, 8]. Most research papers fail to mention the influence of median income. The few reports which did mention it did not report that the direction of influence was different for different age groups. However, the magnitude of the influence of income disparity has been found to be different for different age groups. Lynch and his colleagues have reported that excess mortality associated with disparity was most notable in the elderly[9].

There are several points to be noted in the above-mentioned Japanese analysis. First, the number of prefectures in the study was as small as forty-six (Hyogo Prefecture was excluded due to the damage inflicted on it by the Great Hanshin-Awaji Earthquake Disaster in 1995), making the analysis susceptible to the influence of extreme figures. We must also note that some prefectures have a limited number of samples on which income level/distribution disparity indices were based, making these indices prone to errors. However, we could not solely attribute small sample size and

Table 3.1: Prefectural income distribution, income levels and age-adjusted mortality rates

	Pearson correlation with Gini index	Partial correlation coefficient with Gini index if prefectural median income is included in analysis	Partial correlation coefficient with prefectural median income
Male			
All ages	0.45^b	0.30^b	-0.37^b
0–14	-0.12	0.00	0.24
15–59	0.28^a	-0.01	-0.64^b
≥60	0.10	0.34^b	0.51^b
Female			
All ages	0.35^b	0.35^b	0.07
0–14	0.12	0.04	-0.15
15–59	0.28^a	0.01	-0.59^b
≥60	0.06	0.31^b	0.53^b

Notes. a: $p < 0.10$; b: $p < 0.05$.

Source: Age-adjusted mortality rates are based on the *1995 National Census of Japan and Vital Statistics of Japan*. Prefectural incomes are based on the *1995 Comprehensive Survey of Living Conditions of the People on Health and Welfare*.

potential errors to the difference between previous findings in the USA and ours, because we still found similar patterns across age and gender groups even after excluding extreme prefectural observations with small samples.

Previous US studies were mainly based on the 1990 US National Census. Mellor and Milyo have reported that with the census data in years other than 1990, a significant association between mortality and income disparity was consistently found after controlling for average income level[6]. Nakaya and Dorling conducted a comparative study using census data from the UK and Japan, and demonstrated that the relationship between income and mortality rates differs in different age groups in Japan, but not in the UK[11]. There have been no studies in Japan which analyse time-series cross-sectional data on this issue. However, as the analysis by Nakaya and Dorling (based on 1989 data) and that by us (based on 1995 data) are approximately six years apart, it seems fair to say that there is a consistent and distinct tendency among elderly Japanese: that is, the higher the local income level, the higher the mortality, irrespective of the year of investigation.

As the above discussion shows, previous studies on the ecological association between mortality rates and income levels/distribution across geographical regions have produced more questions than answers. Unfortunately, there is currently an overwhelming lack of reports from countries other than the USA and the UK on more detailed analyses of ecological data. The research circle of social epidemiology has shifted its interest to multilevel analysis rather than ecological studies that are often susceptible to 'ecological fallacy.' However, before jumping into multilevel analysis, researchers should have discussed in depth whether we could assumingly interpret variables such as the 'Gini index' and 'median income level' in a consistent and definite manner across different countries, regions and cultures, and what aspects of economic level are reflected in these variables. There has been a report that even in an analysis of US data, the association between income disparity and mortality rates no longer exists after local medical resources and unemployment rates are corrected for.[12] Another US study of time-series data analysis from 1978 to 2000 has shown the most drastic decrease in mortality rates was found in the region which developed the widest income disparity during the study period[13, 14]. These studies suggest that we should take caution before we interpret the found relationship between a population's health and income disparities too literally, and simply lead them to the political argument concerning the appropriateness of income redistribution. There is a need for further scientific studies to describe various patterns of association between health and income disparity based not only on cross-sectional data, but also on time-series, cross-sectional and multi-regional/national data[15].

Multilevel data analyses

Critique of previous US studies

The conclusion that 'income disparity negatively affects the health of the population', which was found mainly using US state-level data, was met with immediate theoretical criticism[16].

Figure 3.3 shows a hypothetical relationship between an individual's likelihood of early death and his/her income level: the higher the absolute income, the lower the likelihood of early death. The point is that this relationship is not linear but is represented

Figure 3.3: A hypothetical relationship between health status (risk) and income

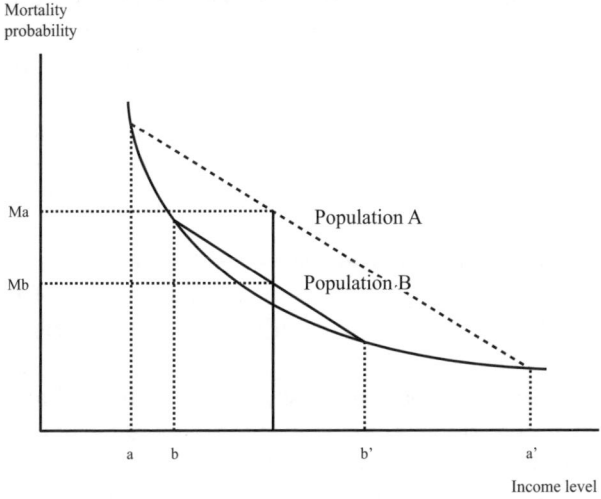

by a concave curve. Let us compare the relationship between income disparity and the mortality rate of two populations, A and B. Suppose that in Population A and Population B the income levels range between a–a' and b–b', respectively. This means that Population A has a wider income disparity. If we calculate the average likelihood of early death in each population, the average figure will be higher in Population A than in Population B because of the curved relationship between individual income level and death risk. This means that a nonlinear relationship between absolute income and death risk at the individual level could explain the population-level relationship between income disparity and mortality rates, as were found in previous studies.

This controversy is still lingering. In their 2004 review, Subramanian and Kawachi used the term 'concavity effects' to describe the apparent effects of income levels caused by a nonlinear relationship as mentioned above. These researchers also proposed to use the term 'pollution effects' to refer to the 'direct' effects (if any) of local income disparity on health, and attempted to distinguish between these two types of effects[17]. The former, concavity effects, are not actually 'indirect'; they provide a clear-cut model of the pathway on how income disparity in a population would result in a lower health level of the population as a whole. In fact, Hugh Gravelle, who was critical of the pollution effects theory, has estimated potential health improvement effects which may be achieved by narrowing the income disparity in a population[18].

The point at issue here is quite theoretical. The problem is whether people's health is affected by the concavity effects, represented by individual income levels, or the pollution effects, represented by the characteristics of the locality or population such as income disparity. This issue has lead to a debate between the 'absolute income hypothesis' and the 'relative income hypothesis' [19]. Unfortunately, this has been misleadingly simplified into the political debate between those who insist on economic growth to raise average income levels, and those who insist on welfare programs for more equal redistribution of income within a population. I will keep my comment on this 'politicization' of studies on health and income until later in this chapter.

Technically speaking, whether or not income distribution (which is a population characteristic) has any effects on people's health cannot be determined without taking into account the confounding effects of individual income levels. Moreover, the analysis would require a statistical method that takes the hierarchical nature of data into consideration (multilevel analysis), instead of a conventional, simple, linear model. These are the very reasons studies on 'multilevel analysis of income disparity' have been published one after another since 1997 [20-28].

All of the studies based on multilevel data published in the late 1990s were reported from the USA, partly due to the availability of large-scale public official data. Strangely, among studies using the same data source, some found 'significant' effects of income disparity, while others failed to do so (Tables 3.2-1 & 3.2-2).

In their review, Subramanian and Kawachi listed the following four points as reasons for the mixed results[17]:
- Treatment of individual income as a variable.
  If income is included in the model as a continuous variable, despite the nonlinear relationship between individual income and health level (or risk), the model could measure only the linear part of the relationship, and the remaining nonlinear part of the relationship might have been picked up falsely by income disparity variables such as the state-level Gini index. This is a point criticised by Gravelle. However, the published studies included income as a dummy variable with four to five levels, and should allow their model to absorb the nonlinear part of the relationship between the income and health.
- Treatment of mean/median local income in the analysis

Most of the multilevel studies published in the USA included in their analytic model only individual income and regional income disparity, and did not include mean or median regional income. There are a few studies which did include mean or median regional income in the analysis, but failed to report the results (these studies usually add simply that the addition of mean regional income produced no change in the results). In their analysis, Blakely and his colleagues reported that the addition of state-level mean income resulted in a loss in significance of the Gini index[25]. The authors concluded that the effects of income disparity which had been reported in previous studies might have been confounded by regional income level. However, they also argued that the inclusion of individual income AND aggregated income variables in the model would result in over-controlling, which would undermine the intrinsic significance of income disparity[19, 25]. Nevertheless, as proposed by Wagstaff and van Doorslaer[32] in their theoretical models of income and health, if we attempt to purify the potential effects of relative position in the population (the position of a person's income relative to the average regional income level), we need to include median/mean income in addition to absolute individual income and income disparity of the population.

- Treatment of regional dummies

One issue which has been debated mainly between Subramanian and Kawachi, and Mellor and Milyo is whether or not to include the fixed effects of the region itself in the model. Mellor and Milyo have pointed out that if the model fails to include sufficient regional variables other than income disparity, the effects of regional characteristics which may have associations with income disparity (such as social/ political culture or social welfare policy/resources which are specific to the region) may be falsely picked up as effects of income disparity. They argue that the potential effects of non-specific regional characteristics should be absorbed by adding regional dummy variables to the model[29]; and clearly, addition of these kinds of dummy variables usually reduces the effects of regional income disparity. On the other hand, Subramanian and his colleague understood this issue as a matter of regional clustering and level-setting. They maintain that three-level multilevel modelling instead of two-level modelling should be used, and to set a greater region above county and state as the third level. They have reported that

Table 3.2-1: A list of studies based on multilevel analysis using US and Japanese data (cross-sectional studies)

Authors	Year published	Ref. No	Data	Sample size	Geographical unit	Individual income	Confounding factors on individual level	Local income level	Income distribution	Regional dummy variables	Statistical method	Effects of income distribution
Kennedy, et al	1998	20	Behavioral Risk Factor Surveillance System (1993, 1994)	205,245	50 States (1,259-8,800 persons/State)	5 levels, uncorrected for number of household members	Age, gender, education, medical insurance status, family composition	Not included	State Gini index calculated from Current Population Survey 1990-1992, categorised into 4 levels.	None	SUDAAN logistic regression	Effects existed.
Soobader and LeClere	1999	21	National Health Interview Survey (1989-1991)	9,637	564 counties (3,642 investigational districts, approx. 4,000 persons/district)	4 levels, uncorrected for number of household members	Age, education, occupation	Median local income, proportion of poor households	Gini index obtained from 1990 National Census data, categorised into 4 levels.	None	SUDAAN logistic regression	Negative effects at county level, not significant at investigational district level.
Subramanian, et al	2001	22	Behavioral Risk Factor Surveillance System (1993, 1994)	144,692	39 States (1,181-7,212 persons/State)	3 levels, uncorrected for number of household members	Age, gender, race, marital status, medical insurance status, smoking status	Median local income	State Gini index, calculated as continuous variables from Current Population Survey 1990-1992.	None	MLwiN logistic regression	Negative effects in the high-income group.
Blakely, et al.	2002	25	Current Population Survey (1995, 1997)	185,479	232 metropolitan areas	4 levels, corrected for number of household members	Age, gender, race	Mean State income (4 levels)	Gini index (obtained from National Census), 0.417+/- 0.025; upper limit, 0.467; categorised into 4 levels.	None	SAS Proc Glimmix (random-intercept model)	Effects disappeared upon inclusion of mean State income.

Income Distribution and Health

Authors	Year published	Ref. No	Data	Sample size	Geographical unit	Individual income	Confounding factors on individual level	Local income level	Income distribution	Regional dummy variables	Statistical method	Effects of income distribution
Mellor and Milyo	2003	29	Current Population Survey (1995-1999)	309,135 (approx. 60,000 persons/ 5 years)	50 States	Continuous variables, uncorrected for number of household members	Age, square of age, race, marital status, medical insurance status, living area, number of household members	Mean State income	State Gini index (for 5, 10 and 20 years from the year of investigation).	Fixed effects	Probit analysis (using robust error estimation)	Significant negative effects existed before, but disappeared after, correction for local fixed effects.
Subramanian and Kawachi	2003	31	Current Population Survey (1995, 1997)	90,006		9 levels, corrected for number of household members	Age, gender, race	Median State income	State Gini index (for 0, 4, 8, 12 and 16 years from the year of investigation)	Comparison by three-layered multilevel analysis (with or without fixed effects of regions)	MLwiN logistic regression	Effects disappeared upon inclusion of fixed effects. Significance achieved in three-layered multilevel analysis.
Shibuya, et al.	2002	30	Comprehensive Survey of Living Conditions of the People on Health and Welfare (1995)	80,899	46 Japanese prefectures (except the earthquake-stricken Hyōgo prefecture)	7 levels, corrected for number of household members	Age, gender, marital status, medical checkup status	Median prefectural income (5 levels)	Prefectural Gini index, categorised into 5 levels.	Fixed effects in 12 regions in the country	SUDAAN logistic regression	Trend (but not significant) toward negative effects.

Note: In all studies, outcome was subjective health levels (dichotomous variables).

Table 3.2-2: A list of studies based on multilevel analysis using US data (longitudinal studies)

Authors	Year published	Ref. No.	Data	Sample size	Geographical unit	Individual income	Confounding factors on individual level	Local income level	Income distribution	Statistical method	Effects of income distribution
Fiscella & Franks	1997	28	National Health and Nutrition Examination Survey (1971-1975)	14,407	Counties (105 districts), 48-323 persons/area)	Continuous variables consisting of medians of 12 categories. Uncorrected.	Age, gender, number of household members	Not included	Continuous variables consisting of ratios of total income earned by people in lower 50 percentile to total income (0.18-0.37).	SUDAAN survival analysis	Not significant
Daly, et al.	1998	27	Panel Study of Income Dynamics (1978 & 1988 cohorts)	6,500?	States (number unknown)	Household income. Details unknown.	Age, gender, race	Median State income	Ratio of total income earned by people in lower 50 percentile to total income, and two other indices. Calculated as continuous variables based on 1980 and 1990 National Censuses	Conventional logistic analysis	Not significant
Lochner, et al.	2001	23	National Health Interview Survey-National Death Index (1987-1995)	546,888	50 States	5 levels categorised by ratio of medians of 27 categories to poverty line. Uncorrected.	Age, gender, race, marital status	Not included	Calculated using State Gini index, poverty ratio and Current Population Survey 1991-1993, and categorised into 5 levels.	SUDAAN survival analysis	Effects existed.

Note: In all studies, outcome was death (obtained from Vital Statistics of the US). None of the above studies includes local dummy variables the effects of income disparity remained significant after the three-level modelling was attempted[17]. I would support Mellor and Milyo's position in this debate because the level-setting in itself would not be effective to counter confounding effects due to region-level covariates.

- Statistical methods

  Finally, there are two types of multilevel statistical methods: a marginal approach using the generalised estimating equations (GEE); and a conditional approach using the random coefficient models. The latter approach explicitly models the variance within/between the regional levels and is able to directly estimate inter-group variance. It is known that in estimating 'fixed effects' of second-level variables such as regional income disparity, these two approaches will produce comparable results if the outcome is a continuous variable. On the other hand, a marginal approach is known to produce a somewhat underestimated regression coefficient if the outcome is binary (good health/poor health)[33]. For this reason, Subramanian and Kawachi have recommended use of the conditional approach. However, the two approaches differ not only in the treatment of intergroup error, but also in the interpretation of obtained regression coefficients because of different assumptions made in the statistical approaches. Thus, we cannot definitely say which statistical approach is better. Rather, as we can see in Tables 3.2-1 & 3.2-2, the manner by which individual-level variables and regional-level variables are selected and incorporated into the analytic model would make a far larger difference across the studies.

A technical caution must be paid to the patterns in the within- and between-region variations when we select statistical models[33-35]. For instance, if the within-region variation is greater than the between-region variation, there is not much point in using a multilevel analysis in the first place. Another example is excessively large between-region variation. If the between-region variation is such that different regions have totally different ranges of variation (e.g. one region has Gini indices of up to 0.3 while another has Gini indices of at least 0.45), it will never be known whether the observed difference reflects the effects of disparity or is simply a regional difference. This holds true particularly for US data. The extreme variations observed in different US regions seem to be one of the reasons for the high incidence of 'significance of income disparity'.

These differences in methodology must definitely be part of the reason for the mixed results of the previous studies on the potential effects of income disparity. However, I would argue that more fundamental is the lack of a valid theory that links income disparity as a regional characteristic and individual health status, and that this in turn weakens the discriminatory power of the models in question. An either-or question of whether or not income disparity has effects on individual health is no longer productive and may not provide a driving force for further advancement of research in this field. In order to elucidate the mechanisms connecting individual health and regional characteristics, higher priority should be given to theoretically understanding the reason why the same data has produced mixed results. It has become ever more necessary to attempt reconstruction of the theory connecting regional socioeconomic characteristics and individual health status. For this purpose, a broader mode of scientific inquiry may be required; we may sincerely get back to the original findings of ecological data, and we may want to use qualitative research as well, before boldly jumping into statistical techniques without proper theoretical grounds.

Findings from Japanese studies

For comparison, results of our own study based on Japanese public data are shown in the last line of Table 3.2-1. This study is often cited as counter-evidence showing that there is no effect of income disparity on health in egalitarian societies such as Japan, in contrast to the USA[36]. However, this was not what we meant. Unfortunately, our study was caught up in the either-or debate of whether or not income disparity has effects on health. In this section, I would like to provide some supplementary explanations and discussion of this study.

Our analysis was based on several hypotheses:
1. What is reflected in the Gini index is probably not income disparity itself; the observed association was contaminated by a confounding bias due to the individual-level association between income and health status. The Gini index must also be characterised as an 'approximate' variable which reflects differences in regional characteristics from which disparities arise. Examples of these regional characteristics include economic and industrial structures, socio-political cultures, as well as social, welfare and economic policies, and cultural attitudes toward disparities.

2. If the above hypothesis is correct, a model including the Gini index only would find a significant association between the index and health. Addition of individual income to this model would markedly reduce the effect of the Gini index on health. The effect of the Gini index would be further reduced by inclusion in the model of regional dummy variables in order to absorb the non-specific differences in regional characteristics.
3. Any effect of the Gini index remaining after these procedures must be pinned down, including the potential effect of economic disparity.

We tested the above hypotheses with hierarchical modelling as shown in Table 3.3. The results supported our hypotheses. The univariate model found 'income disparity' to be a significant factor: the wider the income disparity in the region where a person lived, the higher, in a dose-dependent manner, were the odds of an answer that he/she was in poor health. The addition of 'median regional income' to this model (Model 1), followed by the addition of 'individual income' and other individual-level variables (Model 2), resulted in a loss of significance of 'income disparity'. At this stage, the dose-response relationship was no longer observed. In point estimation, the consistent trend no longer existed, as seen in the tendency that regions with wider disparities were likely to have people in better health. However, at this stage the trend remained that the higher the mean prefectural income, the lower the 'poor health' odds. Finally, when we added the dummy variables for twelve regional blocks in order to absorb non-specific regional characteristics (Model 3), two points emerged:

- Although failing to reach significance, the trend reappeared, namely, that the odds of poor health were higher in the fourth quartile of the Gini index (the category of the widest income disparity); and
- The direction of the effect of median income was reversed; there was a linear trend, namely, that the higher the median income for the region in which a person lived, the more likely he/she reported poor health.

Unfortunately, the paper published in the *British Medical Journal* skipped explaining this hierarchical modelling. The full paper made available on the website also omitted some details. This has resulted in our findings being quoted, against our will, in support of the conclusion that no effect of income disparity on health was observed in Japan[30]. If asked whether there is any relationship between the Gini

Table 3.3: An analysis of data from a 1995 Comprehensive Survey of Living Conditions of the People on Health and Welfare (N = 80899) (modified from Shibuya, et al. 2002)

	Univariate model		Model 1		Model 2		Model 3	
	Odds ratio	(95% CI)	Odds ratio	(95% CI)	Odds ratio	(95% CI)	Odds ratio	(95% CI)
Gini index								
1st quartile	1.00		1.00		1.00		1.00	
2nd quartile	1.00	(0.92–1.10)	0.97	(0.89–1.07)	1.00	(0.91–1.11)	0.99	(0.89–1.11)
3rd quartile	1.07	(0.98–1.18)	1.03	(0.94–1.14)	1.03	(0.93–1.14)	1.02	(0.90–1.17)
4th quartile	1.14	(1.02–1.27)	0.90	(0.78–1.05)	0.90	(0.77–1.04)	1.13	(0.96–1.34)
Median prefectural income								
1st quartile	1.33	(1.20–1.47)	1.39	(1.22–1.58)	1.14	(1.01–1.30)	0.79	(0.64–0.99)
2nd quartile	1.15	(1.07–1.24)	1.13	(1.03–1.23)	1.03	(0.94–1.13)	0.85	(0.71–1.01)
3rd quartile	1.15	(1.05–1.25)	1.11	(1.01–1.22)	1.03	(0.94–1.14)	0.93	(0.83–1.04)
4th quartile	1.00		1.00		1.00		1.00	

Note: Model 1 includes the Gini index and median prefectural income only. Model 2 includes the variables in Model 1 plus individual-level variables (age, gender, individual income, marital status and medical checkup status). Model 3 includes the variables in Model 2 plus regional dummy variables (a total of twelve blocks nationwide).

Source: http://bmj.bmjjournals.com/cgi/reprint/324/7328/116

index and the subjective health of individuals in the Japanese data, the answer is 'yes'. If the Gini index is added as a continuous variable, there is a 'significant' negative relationship with subjective health status[37]. The point is whether we should then jump to the conclusion that 'income disparity has a negative effect on health', or take a more prudent attitude based on theoretical considerations.

Our points of discussion were: 1) Why was the observed effect of income disparity not as strong as that in the USA? 2) How should we interpret the behaviour of 'median income' before and after the inclusion of regional variables? 3) How should we interpret the remaining effect of the Gini index? In relation to the first point, the gap in the degree of income disparity between Japan and the USA has often been mentioned. It is true that the US national Gini index for 1995–1997 was reported to be 0.4225, which is higher than the 1995 Japanese counterpart number of 0.36. However, if the USA simply had a wider income disparity as a whole, it would not necessarily lead to a positive finding of the effect of regional income disparity across states. Only when the degree of income disparity between regions had a large variance, should we be able to extract the effects of the income disparity. A recent international comparative study[38, 39] conducted an analysis of multilevel data collected from regional units located in US and Canadian metropolitan areas. When only Canadian samples were used, income disparity was not found to be significant, while addition of US samples resulted in a positive finding of income disparity effect. The US samples contained both the regions with minimum disparity and maximum disparity. The reason income disparity tends to be significant in the analyses of US data may just be because the USA has a wide between-region income disparity (a wide disparity between equal regions and unequal regions), rather than having a wide income disparity as a whole. This kind of effect may be easily detected in the USA, whose states have their own distinctive constitutions and government frameworks. In other words, even if income disparity has an effect on health in Japan or Canada, researchers may have been unable to detect the effect because of these countries' narrower between-region disparities.

Concerning the second discussion point (the behaviour of median income), Soobader and LeClere,[21] and Blakely, Lochner and Kawachi[25] come to the same conclusion: including mean or median income in the model results in a reduction of the effect of income disparity. Strangely, on the other hand, our finding that inclusion of the regional dummy variables resulted in a reversal of the effect of mean income is shared by Mellor and Milyo's results[29]. We should be very cautious to take this as a universal phenomenon, as Mellor and Milyo's study and ours are the only ones which expressly included regional dummy variables in the model. In our case, we inferred from the finding that the 'relative position of a person's income in the region' expressed as 'individual income minus standard regional income' may have an effect on his/her subjective health status, instead of concluding that a 'high regional income level has a negative effect on health'. It is intriguing that this phenomenon was observed only when non-specific regional differences were absorbed by inclusion of the regional dummy variables. It is difficult to advance this argument further as, unfortunately, there have been no other studies that expressly discuss 'relative income level'[19]. We later analysed whether this phenomenon is more commonly observed, using data from other years. The results showed that this phenomenon was uniquely found only in the 1995 data[37]. The effect of mean income significantly differed between different years and between different age groups (unpublished data).

With respect to the third issue – the effect of the Gini index remaining after the inclusion of the regional dummy variables – it is debatable whether this remaining effect should be interpreted as truly representing the 'effect of income disparity on health'. Assuming that a wide income disparity is associated with an unequal society and a lack of social capital (as argued by Kawachi and Kennedy[40]), it is puzzling that the effect of a wide income disparity is more prominent at the county or state level rather than at the smaller district level, which is closer and more relevant to social comparison between individual citizens. We could not test how the different levels of aggregation affect the study findings because the sampling strategy of the Japanese public data did not allow us to calculate income distribution indices for a level below prefecture. However, it is unlikely at least theoretically that prefectural income disparity would reflect the prefectural disparity in social capital. It would be more natural to think that the remaining effect of the Gini index reflects the differences in economic structure and social welfare policy between different regions as political units, whether they are states, prefectures or regional blocks[6, 15].

Time-series studies

Both the cross-sectional studies and the longitudinal studies shown in Tables 3.2-1 and 3.2-2, respectively, use income disparity at one point in time as the exposure factor. In either case, analysis of income disparity is subject to the effects of unmeasured confounding factors, because whether or not a person lives in a certain region where the disparity exists is determined not at random, but by some kind of selection process. This is an issue of so-called 'confounding by indication'. Economic and other studies have used the instrumental variable method and other similar methods as ways of overcoming this type of selection problem, though such methods have not yet been utilized in the field of social epidemiology. Some social epidemiologists even hold an extremely pessimistic opinion that no observational studies would be able to elucidate this issue, and insist on social experiments as the only solution[41].

There are some natural-experimental situations (such as reinforced redistribution due to a policy change) that would allow researchers to use a quasi-experimental approach, such as time-series analysis. The study by Mellor and her colleague[6, 29] is a good example of this. They analysed US time-series cross-sectional data. They have shown that income disparities have in fact widened in regions with decreased mortality rates over time, a finding which opposes the income disparity hypothesis. Another example is a study from Taiwan. Chiang[42] reported that during the 1970s, the period preceding Taiwan's rapid economic growth, mortality rates had a strong association with absolute income levels. In contrast, during the 1980s, which is the post-rapid growth period, mortality rates had a stronger association with the Gini index. This is in line with the relative income hypothesis. Also, using Israeli time-series cross-sectional data from 1979–2000, Shmueli[43] conducted an analysis of the relationship between the changes in average life expectancy and mortality rates and the changes in GDP and the Gini index. Shmueli showed that while the income disparity itself increased, the national health level improved as a result of a reinforced income redistribution policy.

We have also attempted a time-series cross-sectional analysis of data from the Japanese Comprehensive Survey of Living Conditions of the People on Health and Welfare in the period 1986–1998 [37]. During the late 1980s through to the 1990s, the Japanese economy experienced a period of upheaval, from the height of the bubble economy to the first negative growth since the end of World War II. During this period, real income levels as well as nominal income levels improved, and the Gini index increased from 0.33 to 0.36. We analysed the association of subjective health status with individual incomes, median regional incomes, and regional Gini indices. The results showed a strong and positive association between individual income and health, though the magnitude of the effect differed significantly across gender and marital status. Median income showed a negative association with self-reported health for 1995 only, with the data from all other years failing to show any significant trends. The effect of median income also significantly differed depending on age and birth cohort. As expected, the Gini index, treated as a continuous variable, showed a significant negative association with health status. However, it showed no significant interaction with any of the covariates, including age, birth cohort, gender and marital status, or with the year of survey. This means that income disparity showed no interaction with individual characteristics, nor with the economic changes over time, whilst the impact of income disparity would predictably be different in different layers of socioeconomic status and in different economic environments. This fails to support the hypothesis that income disparity causes psychological stress arising from social comparison, as Kawachi and his colleagues supposed.[49] We then concluded again that it would be more natural to argue that the Gini index represents a fixed effect reflecting a community's socio-political/industrial characteristics, rather than an index of economic inequality per se.

Hypotheses for how income distribution and health connect

I have thus far provided an outline of the studies which have analysed the relationship between socioeconomic conditions and health, focusing on income disparity. By what mechanism then, does income disparity affect health?

A primary potential mechanism is the materialistic one. Called 'neo-materialism' by some, this is the view that the absolute amount of resources allocated to education, medical services, welfare and other services affects health. This view holds that a community with a wide disparity would show a difference in health status between the wealthy class, having strong political and economic power, and the rest of the community who have less. Specifically, when the resources allocated to relatively poor classes are very small, disparity would have a negative effect on their health. If this view were correct, the effect of disparity would be more apparent in poorer classes, and indeed, there have been reports supporting this view.

A second potential mechanism is the behavioural one. It is argued that belonging to different social classes leads to different lifestyle behaviours which in turn, lead to different patterns of disease occurrence. One study has shown a strong association between income/education and lifestyle behaviours, such as smoking, eating habits and exercise[45]. Some have also argued that different lifestyle behaviours in different classes arise from inequality of education, resources and opportunities, while others have argued that they arise from different preferences and cultures in different classes.

A third potential mechanism is social comparison. This view holds that each person belongs to a community which has its own mode and standard of living[46, 47], and failure to comply with this mode or to reach this standard can cause psychological stress in the person, eventually leading to disease or poorer health[48].

A fourth hypothesis that has attracted attention is that stress caused by a lack of social capital affects health. For the definition of social capital and related studies, readers should refer to the chapter by Katsunori Kondō. There has been a study supporting this hypothesis, although indirectly[49].

There has been no integrated grand theoretical framework for comparing and verifying these alternative hypotheses, and supporters of respective hypotheses seem to have done little more than dispute each other's views. What we need to advance in this field of study is a new theoretical framework, and research that comprehensively includes a variety of intermediate explanatory variables to discriminate between the alternative hypotheses, and that allows the use of more advanced statistical approaches, such as econometric selection models. Particularly, in addition to individual household income, regional income level and regional income disparity, we need an ecological framework of data including individual data on health-related behaviour, self-efficacy and other health beliefs, data on households encompassing individuals (e.g. income and asset resources, informal care capacity and other family support), and data on socio-environmental resources (formal resources from public institutions and environmental safety, and informal resources, such as trust of one's neighbours).

Conclusion

This chapter has provided an outline of ecological and multilevel studies conducted in Japan and elsewhere on the potential association between regional income distribution and health status. As mentioned above, although various approaches have been attempted, it would be fair to say that more questions than answers arise on whether or not any effect exists, the size of the potential effect, and the mechanism by which the effect may be produced. However, researchers seem to have reached a consensus, theoretically and empirically, on the fact that a population with a wide income disparity has poorer health status than a population without a wide income disparity. However, why is this the case? What are the mechanisms involved? What actually are the 'regional characteristics which affect health' represented by the index of regional income distribution? How much do they affect health? Which layer of a community or society is most vulnerable to the effect? In order to answer these questions, it would be necessary to take a comprehensive approach, including development of a methodology to compensate for the weaknesses of traditional observational cross-sectional studies, and introduction of semi-experimental methods of study; or we may have to get back to ecological studies and conduct qualitative research to deepen our understanding of this social phenomenon and reach a new sociological theory in a 'grounded' manner. We may also need to (re)construct the concepts of measurement of 'socioeconomic status,' 'social relationships,' or 'social inequality.' But most fundamental to solving this scientific inquiry of income distribution and health would be, I argue, that we should NOT reduce it too narrowly to the issue of 'inequality and health'. Rather, a breakthrough will be found when we see this issue in a wider and more original research context, in which characteristics of a society and the health of individuals are affected and affect each other. In this sense, research into income distribution and health might have just reached a new starting point.

Literature

1 Wilkinson, R. G. (1992), 'Income distribution and life expectancy', *British Medical Journal*, 304 (6820), pp. 165–168.
2 Men, T., P. Brennan, P. Boffetta and D. Zaridze (2003), 'Russian mortality trends for 1991–2001: analysis by cause and region', *British Medical Journal*, 327 (7421), p. 964.
3 Kariya, T. (2001), *Kaisō-ka Nippon to kyōiku kiki – fubyōdō sai seisan kara iyoku kakusa shakai e* (Education in crisis and stratified Japan: from the reproduction of inequality to an 'incentive divide' society), Tokyo: Yūshindō.
4 Tachibanaki, T. (1998), *Nihon no keizai kakusa – shotoku to shisan kara kangaeru* (Economic disparities in Japan – consideration from income and assets aspects), Tokyo: Iwanami Shoten.
5 Judge, K. (1995), 'Income distribution and life expectancy: a critical appraisal', *British Medical Journal*, 311 (7015), pp. 1282–1285; discussion 1285–1287.
6 Mellor, J. M. and J. Milyo (2001), 'Reexamining the evidence of an ecological association between income inequality and health', *Journal of Health Politics, Policy and Law*, 26 (3), pp. 487–522.
7 Kennedy, B. P., I. Kawachi and D. Prothrow-Stith (1996), 'Income distribution and mortality: cross sectional ecological study of the Robin

hood index in the United States', *British Medical Journal*, 312 (7037), pp. 1004–1007.
8. Kaplan, G. A., E. R. Pamuk, J. W. Lynch, R. D. Cohen and J. L. Balfour (1996), 'Inequality in income and mortality in the United States: analysis of mortality and potential pathways', *British Medical Journal*, 312 (7037), pp. 999–1003.
9. Lynch, J. W., G. A. Kaplan, E. R. Pamuk, R. D. Cohen, K. E. Heck, J. L. Balfour and I. H. Yen (1998), 'Income inequality and mortality in metropolitan areas of the United States', *American Journal of Public Health*, 88 (7), pp. 1074–1080.
10. Yano, E. (2000), 'Hōkatsu teki shihyō ni yoru chiiki no kenkō jōtai no hyōka to sono riyō ni kansuru kenkyū (A study on the assessment of regional health status using comprehensive indices and their use)', *Heisei 11 nendo kōsei kagaku kenkyū hi hojo kin (tōkei jōhō kōdo riyō kenkyū jigyō) hōkoku sho* [FY1999 health sciences research grant (statistical information advanced utilisation research project) report].
11. Nakaya, T. and D. Dorling (200v5), 'Geographical inequalities of mortality by income in two developed island countries: a cross-national comparison of Britain and Japan', *Social Science and Medicine*, 60 (12), pp. 2865–2875.
12. Shi, L., J. Macinko, B. Starfield, J. Xu, and R. Politzer (2003), 'Primary care, income inequality, and stroke mortality in the United States: a longitudinal analysis, 1985–1995', *Stroke*, 34 (8), pp. 1958–1964.
13. Lynch, J., G. D. Smith, S. Harper and M. Hillemeier (2004), 'Is income inequality a determinant of population health? Part 1. A systematic review', *The Milbank Quarterly*, 82 (1), pp. 5–99.
14. Lynch, J., G. D. Smith, S. Harper and M. Hillemeier (2004), '"Is income inequality a determinant of population health? Part 2. U.S. National and regional trends in income inequality and age-and cause-specific mortality', *The Milbank Quarterly*, 82 (2), pp. 355–400.
15. Blakely, T. A. and A. J. Woodward (2000), 'Ecological effects in multi-level studies', *Journal of Epidemiology and Community Health*, 54 (5), pp. 367–374.
16. Gravelle, H. (1998), 'How much of the relation between population mortality and unequal distribution of income is a statistical artefact?', *British Medical Journal*, 316 (7128), pp. 382–385.
17. Subramanian, S.V. and I. Kawachi (2004), 'Income inequality and health: what have we learned so far?', *Epidemiologic Reviews*, 26, pp. 78–91.
18. Gravelle, H. and M. S. Sutton (2003), 'Income related inequalities in self assessed health in Britain: 1979–1995', *Journal of Epidemiology and Community Health*, 57 (2), pp. 125–129.
19. Kawachi, I., S. V. Subramanian and N. Almeida-Filho (2002), 'A glossary for health inequalities', *Journal of Epidemiology and Community Health*, 56 (9), p. 647.
20. Kennedy, B. P., I. Kawachi, R. Glass and D. Prothrow-Stith (1998), 'Income distribution, socioeconomic status, and self rated health in the United States: multilevel analysis', *British Medical Journal*, 317 (7163), pp. 917–921.
21. Soobader, M.-J. and F. B. LeClere (1999), 'Aggregation and the measurement of income inequality: effects on morbidity', *Social Science and Medicine*, 48 (6), pp. 733–744.

22 Subramanian, S.V., I. Kawachi and B. P. Kennedy (2001), 'Does the state you live in make a difference? Multilevel analysis of self-rated health in the US', *Social Science and Medicine*, 53 (1), pp. 9–19.
23 Lochner, K., E. R. Pamuk, D. Makuc, B. P. Kennedy and I. Kawachi (2001), 'State-level income inequality and individual mortality risk: a prospective, multilevel study', *American Journal of Public Health, 91 (3), pp. 385–391.*
24 LeClere, F. B. and M.-J. Soobader (2000), 'The effect of income inequality on the health of selected US demographic groups', *American Journal of Public Health*, 90 (12), pp. 1892–1897.
25 Blakely, T. A., K. Lochner and I. Kawachi (2002), 'Metropolitan area income inequality and self-rated health – a multi-level study', *Social Science and Medicine*, 54 (1), pp. 65–77.
26 Blakely, T. A., B. P. Kennedy, R. Glass and I. Kawachi (2000), 'What is the lag time between income inequality and health status?', *Journal of Epidemiology and Community Health*, 54 (4), pp. 318–319.
27 Daly, M. C., G. J. Duncan, G. A. Kaplan and J. W. Lynch (1998), 'Macro-to-micro links in the relation between income inequality and mortality', *The Millbank Quarterly*, 76 (3), pp. 315–339, 303–304.
28 Fiscella, K. and P. Franks (1997), 'Poverty or income inequality as predictor of mortality: longitudinal cohort study', *British Medical Journal*, 314 (7096), pp. 1724–1727.
29 Mellor, J. M. and J. Milyo (2003), 'Is exposure to income inequality a public health concern? Lagged effects of income inequality on individual and population health', *Health Services Research*, 38 (1p1) pp. 137–151.
30 Shibuya, K., H. Hashimoto and E. Yano (2002), 'Individual income, income distribution, and self rated health in Japan: cross sectional analysis of nationally representative sample', *British Medical Journal*, 324 (7328), pp. 16–19.
31 Subramanian, S.V. and I. Kawachi (2003), 'The association between state income inequality and worse health is not confounded by race', *International Journal of Epidemiology*, 32, pp. 1022–1028.
32 Wagstaff, A. and E. van Doorslaer (2000), 'Income inequality and health: what does the literature tell us?', *Annual Review of Public Health*, 21, pp. 543–567.
33 Diez-Roux, A. V. (2000), 'Multilevel analysis in public health research', *Annual Review of Public Health*, 21, pp. 171–192.
34 Diez-Roux, A. V. (2002), 'A glossary for multilevel analysis', Journal of *Epidemiology and Community Health*, 56 (8), pp. 588–594.
35 Diez-Roux, A. V. (2004), 'The study of group-level factors in epidemiology: rethinking variables, study designs, and analytical approaches', *Epidemiologic Reviews*, 26, pp. 104–111.
36 Marmot, M. G. and G. D. Smith (1989), 'Why are the Japanese living longer?', *British Medical Journal*, 299 (6715), pp. 1547–1551.
37 Hashimoto, H., 'Keizai kakusa ni yoru kenkō eikyō no nenji hendō: kokumin seikatsu kiso chōsa no kaiseki kekka kara (Annual changes in the effect of economic disparity on health: from analysis of the results of Japanese Comprehensive Survey of Living Conditions of the People on Health and Welfare)', presented at the workshop, 'Shakai ekigaku (Social

epidemiology)' of the 74th Scientific Meeting of the Nippon Eisei Gakkai (Japanese Society for Hygiene), held in Tokyo on 24 March 2004.
38 Ross, N. A., M. C. Wolfson, J. R. Dunn, J.-M. Berthelot, G. A. Kaplan and J. W. Lynch (2000), 'Relation between income inequality and mortality in Canada and in the United States: cross sectional assessment using census data and vital statistics', *British Medical Journal*, 320 (7239), pp. 898–902.
39 Ross, N. A. and J. W. Lynch (2004), 'Commentary: the contingencies of income inequality and health: reflections on the Canadian experience', *International Journal of Epidemiology*, 33 (2), pp. 318–319.
40 Kawachi, I. and B. P. Kennedy (1999), 'Income inequality and health: pathways and mechanisms', *Health Services Research*, 34 (1, Part 2), pp. 215–217.
41 Oakes, J. M. (2004), 'The (mis)estimation of neighbourhood effects: causal inference for a practicable social epidemiology', *Social Science and Medicine*, 58 (10), pp. 1929–1952.
42 Chiang, T.-L. (1999), 'Economic transition and changing relation between income inequality and mortality in Taiwan: regression analysis', *British Medical Journal*, 319 (7218), pp. 1162–1165.
43 Shmueli, A. (2004), 'Population health and income inequality: new evidence from Israeli time-series analysis', *International Journal of Epidemiology*, 33 (2), pp. 311–317.
44 Lynch, J. W., G. D. Smith, G. A. Kaplan and J. S. House (2000), 'Income inequality and mortality: importance to health of individual income, psychosocial environment, or material conditions', *British Medical Journal*, 320 (7243), pp. 1200–1204.
45 Lynch, J. W., G. D. Smith and J. T. Salonen (1997), 'Why do poor people behave poorly? Variation in adult health behaviours and psychosocial characteristics by stages of the socioeconomic lifecourse', *Social Science and Medicine*, 44 (6), pp. 809–819.
46 Dressler, W. W. (1985), 'Psychosomatic symptoms, stress, and modernization: a model', *Culture, Medicine and Psychiatry*, 9 (3), pp. 257–286.
47 Dressler, W. W. (1991), 'Social support, lifestyle incongruity, and arterial blood pressure in a southern black community', *Psychosomatic Medicine*, 53 (6), pp. 608–620.
48 Marmot, M. G. and R. G. Wilkinson (2001), 'Psychosocial and material pathways in the relation between income and health: a response to Lynch et al.', *British Medical Journal*, 322 (7296), pp. 1233–1236.
49 Kawachi, I., B. P. Kennedy, K. Lochner and D. Prothrow-Stith (1997), 'Social capital, income inequality, and mortality', *American Journal of Public Health*, 87 (9), pp. 1491–1498.

4 Access to Health Care and Health
Satoshi Toyokawa

Introduction

In using the term 'access to health care', the goals are the receipt of health care as well as consideration of the state of a health care system and/or the barriers to health care. The first condition for health care access is the availability of health care service. The second condition is that the health care meets the residents' needs and is used by the residents. Only then does access to health care become successful. Any failure to satisfy these conditions results in a failure to access health care (Figure 4.1).

Health care access can be assessed within two dimensions[1]. One dimension represents 'availability', which is the degree of adequate supply of health care. The other dimension represents 'utilisation', which is the degree to which health care is actually used. 'Availability' is assessed by the number of physicians and hospital beds per unit population, the distribution of specialists and so on. Reports from many countries have shown regional disparities in the distribution of health care resources. These disparities are often related to geographic barriers. On the other hand, 'utilisation' of health care, which is the degree of fit between clients and the health system, is often analysed from three points of view: personal barriers, organisational barriers and financial barriers. These barriers are closely related to social disparities and have been the subject of study in social epidemiology.

Improving access to health care and achieving equity of access have been among the main goals of health policies in all countries. This chapter focuses on the relation between access to health care and social disparities, and reviews studies which have analysed health care resources along the dimensions of availability and utilisation, in an attempt to consider various barriers.

Figure 4.1: Conditions for having health care access

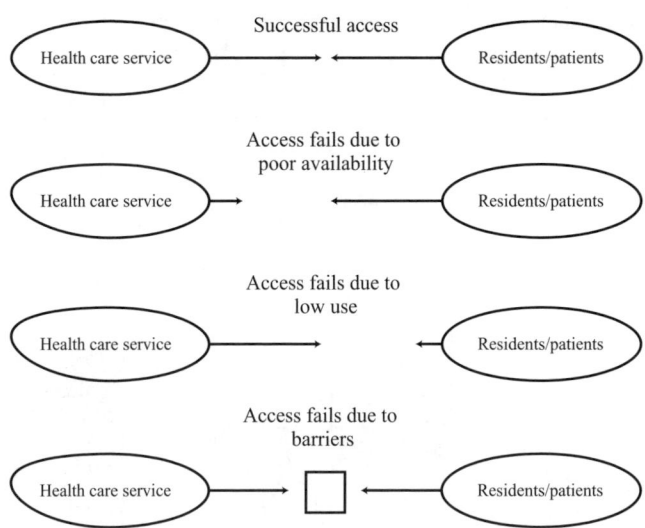

Studies into social disparities and access to health care

Assessment of geographic barriers using GIS

Wang and Luo[2] have analysed the relationship between geographic barriers and socioeconomic barriers to health care access, based on the geographic distribution of physicians in Illinois, USA. Using a geographical information system (GIS), the researchers estimated the travel times between physicians and residents, taking into account the road network and population densities. This estimate was based on the physicians' zip codes and county populations obtained from national census data. Socioeconomic barriers were analysed using socioeconomic variables, socio-cultural variables and health care needs variables, which were all consolidated using factor analysis.

A map showing the variation of geographic accessibility (Figure 4.2) reveals a tendency for cities, including the state's largest city, Chicago, and the state capital, Springfield, to have better spatial access (shown with darker shading) than rural areas (lighter shading). It has been known for impoverished inner-city communities to have poor access to health care, but this is not clear on the accompanying map.

Figure 4.2: Geographical accessibility to primary care

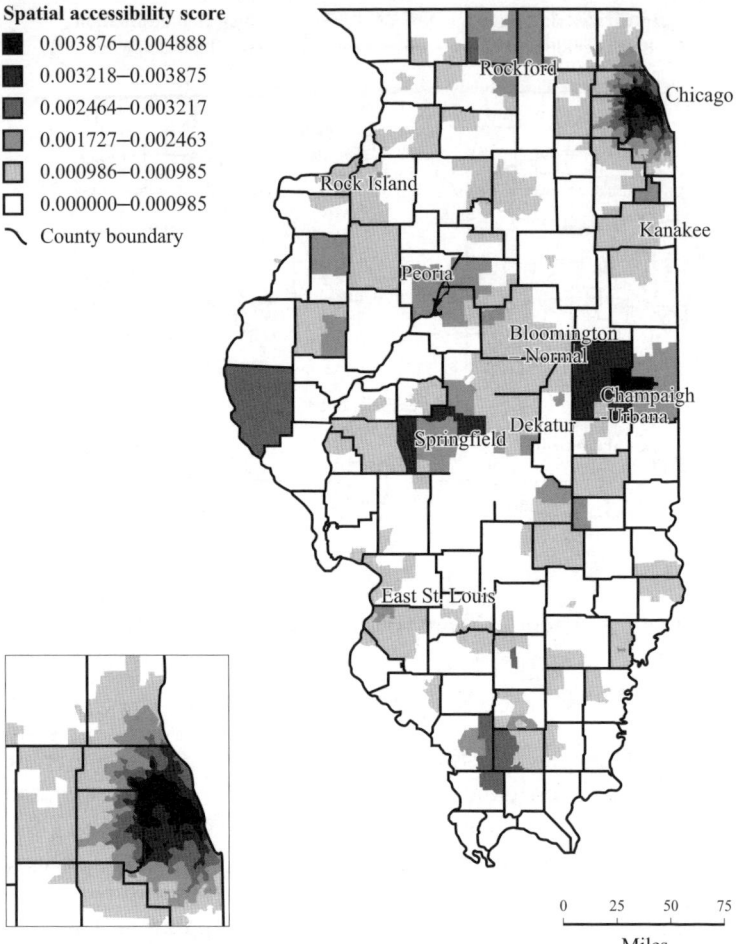

Source: Wang & Luo (2005 p.137)[2]. Reproduced from Figure 3 of the original article with permission from Elsevier.

Figure 4.3 shows maps which identify the distribution of areas of poor health care access based on the results of the socioeconomic barrier assessment. 'Areas of poor spatial access' are tracts in which the absolute number of physicians is low. These areas are agricultural and account for a total of 12.8% of the state's area. The total population in these areas is 215,367 (1.7% of the total state population). Though small in terms of population, these areas

Figure 4.3: Identified physician shortage areas in Illinois, USA

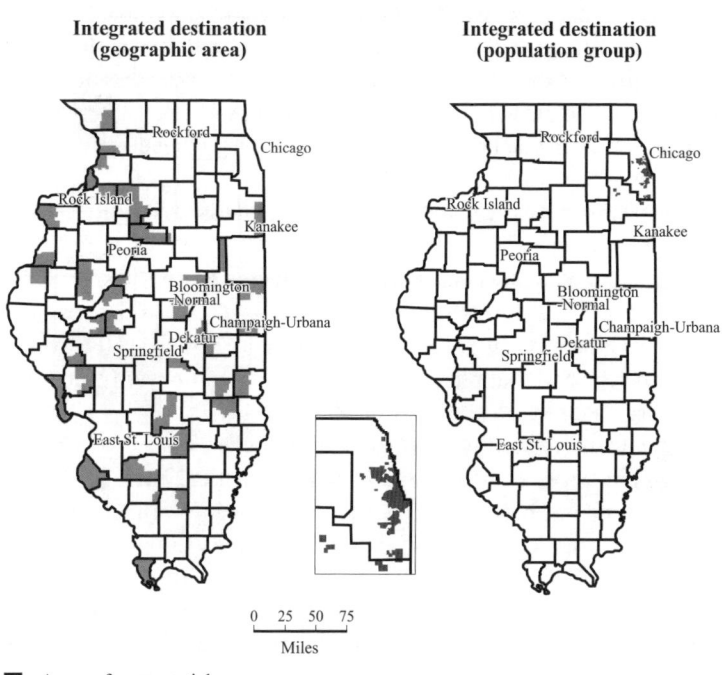

Source: Wang & Luo (2005 p.144) [2]. Reproduced from Figure 7 of the original article with permission from Elsevier.

cover a large proportion of the state's land mass and it is clear that a physician shortage is found mainly in rural areas.

On the other hand, a 'disadvantaged population' is one with poor socioeconomic conditions according to the concept of access to health care. The right-hand map shows that this kind of population is distributed over small areas in cities. It was estimated that the areas with this kind of population account for 0.4% of the state's area and that the total population in these areas is 1,176,085 (9.5% of the total state population). This highlights that health care access is limited due to socioeconomic or socio-cultural conditions mainly in urban areas.

Thus, the association between health care access and social disparities was found to be geographical to such a degree that it can be identified on maps. The use of GIS, which took modes of transportation and other geographical conditions into account, made quantitative analysis possible. This in turn made it possible to assess unequal health care access associated with social disparities. This study highlights that the issue of difficult health care access occurs in both rural and urban areas but for different reasons: the geographical distribution of physicians and social conditions, respectively.

Access to cervical cancer screening and social disparities in Britain

The availability of physicians is a crucial factor for successful health care access. Securing and placing physicians within the reach of patients is a priority in government health care policies. However, it has been reported that physicians are distributed unevenly, and that this is associated with social disparities.

In Britain, it has been shown that there is a geographical association between health and social disparities. For a long time, mortality and morbidity rates have tended to be lower in the southern rather than northern regions, and in rural areas rather than urban areas[3]. Regardless of residents' needs, the availability of health care service has been higher in high income areas and lower in high mortality areas. Julian Tudor Hart used the term 'inverse care law' to describe this distribution of health care service in Britain, and pointed out that the law is more prominently seen in areas subject to market forces[4].

The British health care system is a publicly funded system known as the National Health Service (NHS), under which most health care services are provided at no cost to patients. The NHS has been in place since 1948, and one of its primary objectives was to correct the regional disparities in health care resources. Under the NHS, physicians and hospitals have been allocated to areas without sufficient health services. Meanwhile, areas with sufficient numbers of physicians have not been allotted additional physicians; instead, physicians have been redistributed mainly to deprived areas in cities. However, it has been said that access to specialised or preventive care tends to be improved more slowly in more deprived areas, where access to preventive care is highly necessary but insufficient. It has also been pointed out that the improvement of access to health care has been slow in areas with wide social disparities[5].

Since the reform of the British health care system in 1990, incentives have been provided to each general practitioner who achieves a five-year cervical cancer screening rate of 80% for the residents living in the physician's geographical area of practice. The incidence and mortality rates of cervical cancer have been on the decline since then, which has resulted in screening being well received in Britain. However, the effect of the screening incentives was expected to take longer to spread into deprived areas with high rates of cervical cancer. This prompted Deborah Baker and Elizabeth Middleton to focus on cervical cancer screening and analyse the effect of social disparities on the screening penetration rates, and the incidence and mortality rates of cervical cancer by comparing deprived and affluent areas[6].

Of the ninety-nine district health authorities in Britain, sixty had experienced no district changes. These sixty districts were classified into three categories using the Townsend Deprivation Index: deprived areas, areas that were neither affluent nor deprived, and affluent areas (twenty districts per category). Then the researchers investigated whether the standard screening rate of 80% had been achieved in each health authority.

Most affluent areas had achieved the standard screening rate. However, while the deprived areas had greatly improved screening rates, these rates varied widely between different areas, and many still had not reached 80%. In both types of areas, the screening rates tended to improve significantly between 1991 and 1993 (Figure 4.4).

As for the incidence and mortality rates, both showed declining trends (Figure 4.5). No clear differences were observed in women under 35 years of age, in whom cervical cancer incidence and mortality rates were low. However, considerable reductions in incidence and mortality were observed in women at or above 35 and under 65 in all categories. With incidence rates, greater reductions were seen in deprived areas, while considerable differences remained between different categories. With mortality rates, on which the effect of early detection through screening was expected to be observed, declining trends were observed in all categories. This effect was particularly noticeable in medium-deprivation areas, whose mean screening rate for 1991–1993 was comparable to that for deprived areas, whereas the mean for 1997–1999 was about in the middle of the rates for affluent and deprived areas.

As for the association between incidence/mortality rates and screening rates, in deprived areas, a significant negative association was found between the incidence rate ($r = -0.99$; $P < 0.0012$) and the mortality rate ($r = -0.91$; $p < 0.005$) on the one hand, and on the other, the screening rate in women at or above 35 and under 65 years

Figure 4.4 Distribution of the variable percentage (%) of GPs achieving 80% targets in cervical screening for deprived and affluent areas

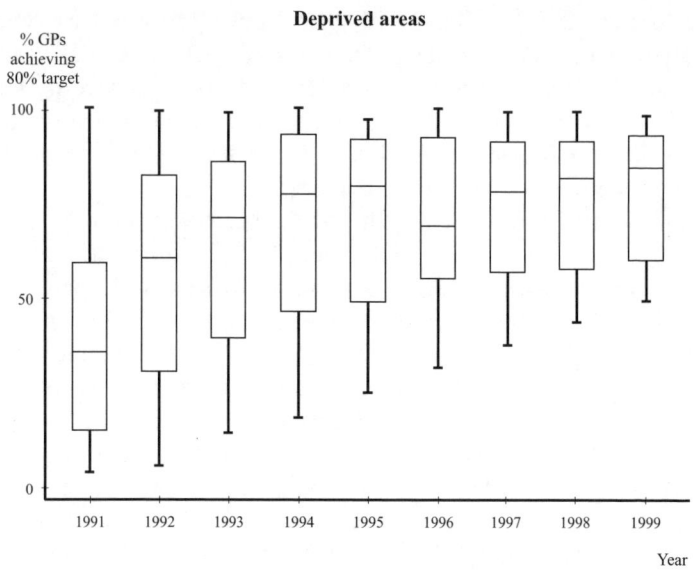

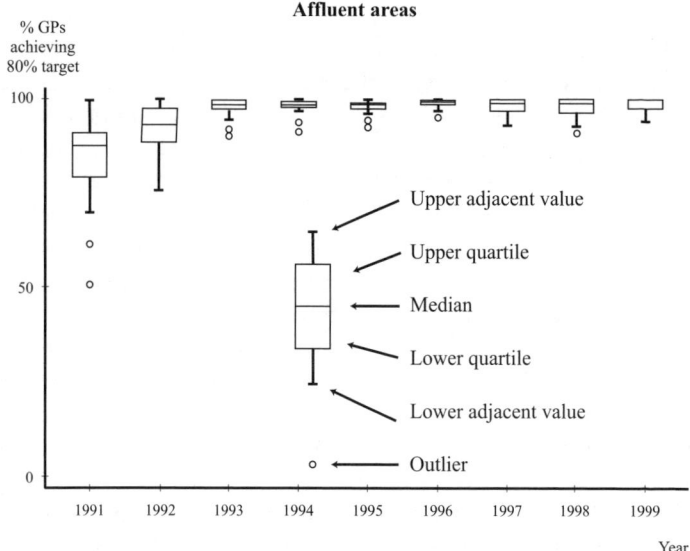

Source: Baker & Middleton (2003)[6]. Reproduced from Figures 1 and 2 of the original article with permission from BMJ Publishing Group.

Figure 4.5: Cervical cancer incidence and mortality rates

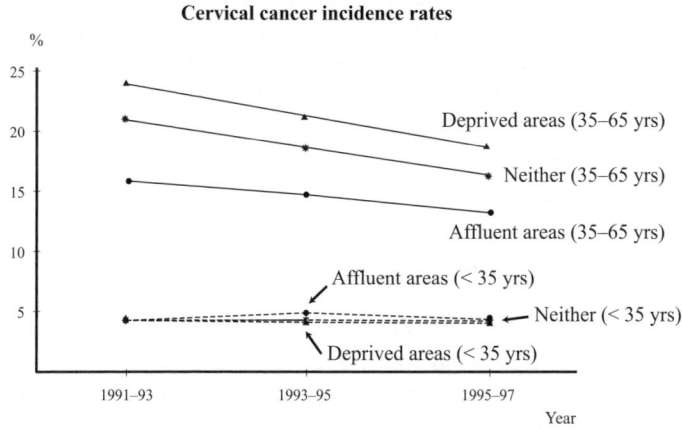

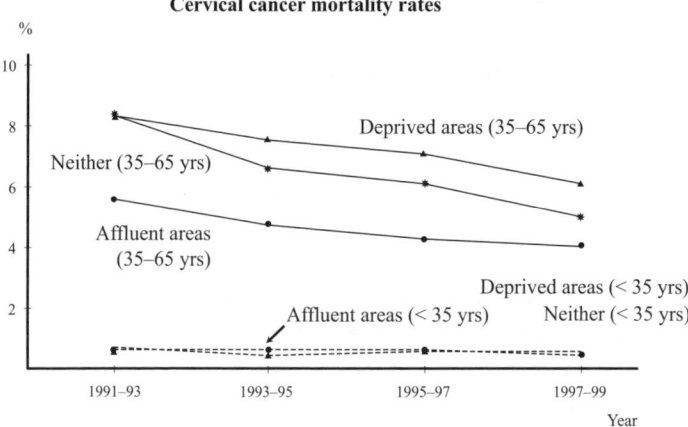

Source: Baker & Middleton (2003)[6]. Created from information from Table 4 of the original article with permission from BMJ Publishing Group.

of age. Similar trends were seen in women below 35 in deprived areas and women in affluent areas, but these associations failed to reach statistical significance.

The spread of screening seems to have resulted first in correcting the inequity in incidence rates, and secondly, in reducing mortality rates toward more comparable rates. The reductions in mortality rates occurred in affluent areas and deprived areas during the first half and the latter half, respectively, of the investigation period.

This may mean that the effect of screening spreads in different ways, depending on different social situations. It has been shown that social disparities constitute a barrier to the spread of the effect of screening incentives. Linking implementation of effective screening with incentives is likely to be effective in narrowing the social disparities in health over the long run. It may be useful to create a situation where the incentives work more effectively in deprived areas.

Despite many reforms of the health care system, it has been reported that physicians distributed in affluent areas in Britain are still about 50% in excess. The uneven distribution of physicians still remains to be improved. In response to the accumulation of these epidemiological findings, the British government has continuously revised relevant standards in order to improve health care access and to reduce social disparities[7].

Assessment of distribution of health care resources

One of the methods of assessing the relationship between income and distribution of health care resources is to use the Lorenz curve with the Gini index[8]. The Lorenz curve is an analytical method devised by the American statistician Conrad Lorenz in 1905, in order to analyse income distribution. It is a curve drawn by plotting in the plane of coordinates the cumulative proportion of population arranged in the order of increasing income (Figure 4.6). First, the cumulative proportion of income earned by people in the lowest 10% income bracket of the population is plotted. The same procedure is repeated for the lowest 20% income bracket. When this procedure is repeated until the total income of the population is plotted, the curve is complete. If the procedure is repeated using short intervals, the curve becomes smooth. If the income distribution is perfectly equal, the Lorenz curve is a straight diagonal line. The Gini index is represented by the area surrounded by the diagonal line and the Lorenz curve. The larger the Gini index, the more unequal the distribution. This technique can be used in many ways. For instance, it can be used to assess the degree of inequality in the distribution of physicians in relation to the population distribution if the vertical axis is replaced with the cumulative proportion of physicians.

Adam Wagstaff and his colleagues conducted an analysis including health care needs in order to assess whether people have access to necessary health care when the need arises[9]. This study uses

Figure 4.6: The Lorenz curve and the Gini index

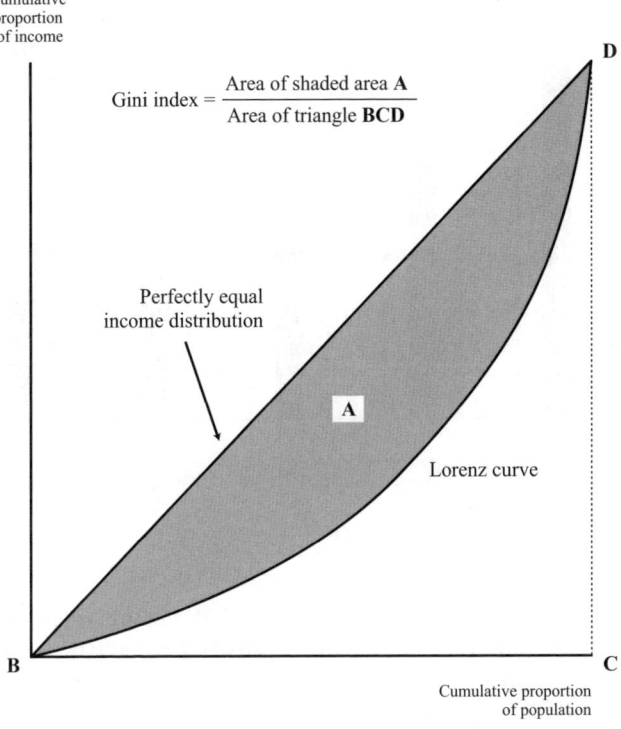

Source: Yamaoka & Kobayashi (1994 p.128)[8].

the Lorenz curve by plotting the disease distribution and medical expenses along the vertical axis to assess the needs and access, respectively. In an analysis of some Dutch data, researchers divided the population into five classes according to income and analysed whether socioeconomic disparities were distributed equally in the distribution of medical expenses (Figure 4.7). The column chart shows that the bottom income class, which accounted for 21% of the population, accounted for more than 31% of the diseases, while accounting for only 27% of the total expenses. A Lorenz curve drawn by plotting the same data shows a separation of the curve of the diseases from that of the medical expenses in lower income brackets, and this disappears in higher income brackets (Figure 4.8). The difference between the two curves assessed quantitatively in terms of area was 0.05. The result of the same analysis conducted for Italian data was 0.11. The larger figure for

Figure 4.7: Expenditure and illness shares, Netherlands 1981–1982

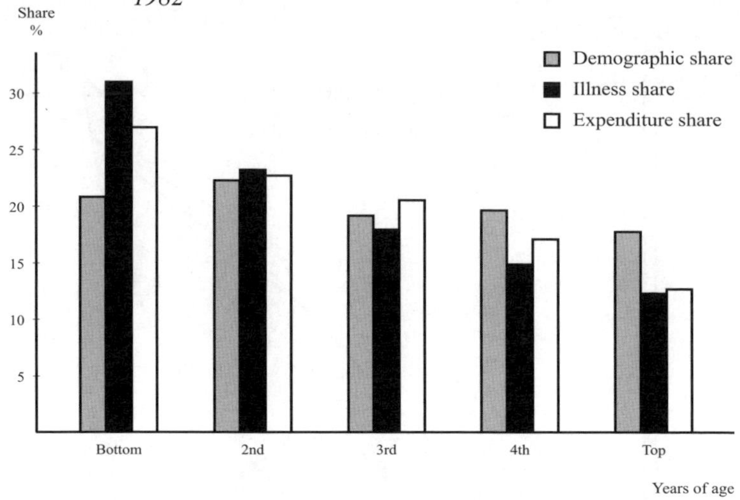

[Bar chart showing Demographic share, Illness share, and Expenditure share across age groups: Bottom, 2nd, 3rd, 4th, Top. Y-axis: Share %. X-axis: Years of age.]

Source: Figure 8 from Wagstaff, van Doorslaer & Paci (1991)[9].

Italy means that the inequality in the balance between medical expense distribution and health status is stronger there than in the Netherlands.

Access to health care can be assessed quantitatively by focusing on the distribution of health care resources. This eventually leads to identification of any unequal distribution, which reflects social disparities. Although this approach does not identify any barrier to health care access, it is a useful method for assessing the availability of health care and social disparities.

Price sensitivity and social disparities in drug consumption

Rising medical expenses covered by health insurance have become a problem worldwide. Countries have increased user charges in the hope of reducing unnecessary medical care. However, there has been some concern that this measure may restrain necessary medical care as well, or may increase social disparities.

In Sweden in 1998, the user charge rate for prescription drugs was 20%. Drug expenses had increased by 133% between 1974 and 1995, which prompted an argument for curbing drug expenses. Most of the drug expenses were prescription drug costs. This led

Figure 4.8: Illness and expenditure concentration curves, Netherlands 1981–1982

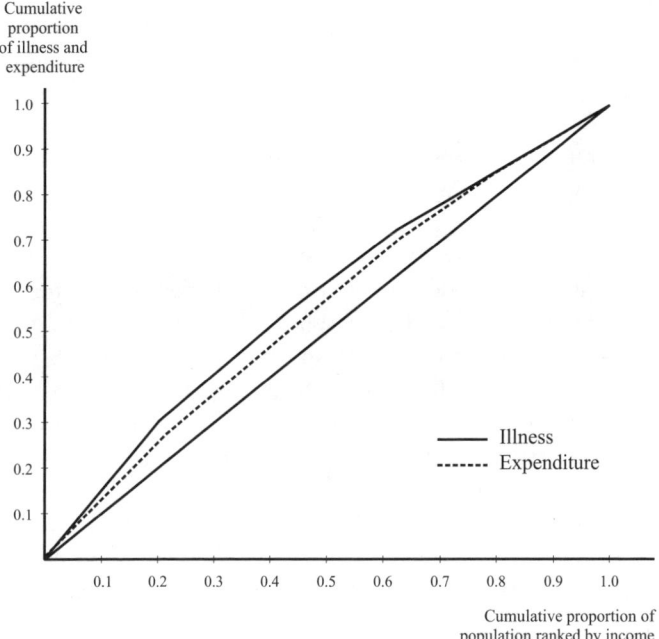

to the argument that user charges for drugs should be increased as a means of holding back the rise in drug expenses.

An increase in the user charge rate for drugs is expected to result in decreased purchases of less effective drugs. This will highlight the price sensitivity of each kind of drug; and the price sensitivity is expected to be affected by social disparities. Lena Lundberg and her colleagues conducted a study to examine the effects of social disparities on the price sensitivity of prescription drugs in the context of changes in user charges[10].

From the questionnaires collected by mail, the data from 2008 eligible respondents were used for analysis. The questionnaires asked the respondents whether an increase in the user charge rate would cause them to refrain from purchasing the prescription drugs they had bought during the preceding six months, assuming that their health status remained the same as during the previous six months. The participants were requested to provide responses to five different rates of user charge increase: 9%, 25%, 56%, 88% or

150%. The statistical model included age, gender, income, education, employment status, self-reported health status and so on.

Seventeen kinds of drugs were analysed, including antihypertensive agents and cough suppressants. In addition to the effects of an increase in user charges, the status of use of the drugs during the previous two weeks was investigated.

In the analysis using multiple logistical regression (Table 4.1), a positive β value means a majority of the respondents answered that they would refrain from purchasing the drug. That is, a higher β value indicated a higher price sensitivity. Analysis of income showed that the higher the income, the smaller the proportion of people who would refrain from purchase: in other words, the higher the income, the lower the price sensitivity was. Thus, an increase of the user charge rate may affect lower income brackets. Similarly, analysis of education levels showed that the higher the education level was, the lower the price sensitivity. Other results show lower price sensitivity in older people, women and people with good self-reported health status.

The analysis of different kinds of drugs showed the lowest price sensitivity in antipyretic/analgesic agents, followed by menopause drugs. The highest price sensitivity was found for cough suppressants, reflecting their low necessity.

An increase in user charges was thus expected to widen the health disparities, through social disparities, such as differences in income or education level. In other words, economic barriers are likely to amplify social disparities.

RAND Health Insurance Experiment

It was believed that an increase in the user charge rate would reduce unnecessary consultation on the one hand, but would, on the other hand, restrict necessary consultation as well. A demonstration of the restrictive effect of a rate increase would require a study which assigns members of the general population to different stepwise user charge rates, and compares their access to health care. It is difficult to conduct this kind of intervention study. Researchers are usually limited to observational studies which compare the situation before and after a certain actual or assumed change in the system. Nonetheless, an intervention study which randomly assigned members of the general population to different charge rates was conducted in the USA[11].

This intervention study, known as the RAND Health Insurance Experiment, was conducted by a private think-tank, the RAND Institute. The study subjects were randomly sampled from six districts located in different parts of the USA. In the study, there were a total of 2,756 households and 7,706 subjects. The study period ran from 1974 to 1982 and was on an extremely large-scale, with the total research expenses amounting to US$60 million at the time. Households whose income was $25,000 (as of 1973) and elderly people were excluded from the study. 15% of all households invited to participate in the study refused to do so.

The households which agreed to participate in the study were randomly assigned to four medical insurance groups whose respective user charge rates were 0% (i.e. free health care), 20%, 50% and 95%. Depending on income, households were assigned to a 5%, 10% or 15% upper limit of user charge. Further, the maximum user charge borne by each household was not to exceed $1,000 a year. Any user charge in excess of this limit was paid by medical insurance. Within the 95% charge rate group, a subgroup was established which was subject to additional upper limits of user charges. In this subgroup, in-patient care was free of charge. For out-patient care, any user charges in excess of $150 per year for any household member or in excess of $450 per year for the entire household were to be paid by medical insurance. As the maximum user charges were thus set on an individual basis, this subgroup was named 'individual deductible' and was characterised by a high likelihood of the participants' user charges exceeding the upper limits. In addition, subsidies were paid to participating households regardless of their use of health care services in order to ensure that their participation in the experiment would not adversely impact on their financial situation because of potential increases in premium payments or otherwise.

Table 4.2 shows the percentages of participants who used health care services in the groups with different user charge rates. The results show that the higher the user charge rate, the smaller the percentage of participants who used health care service. It was also shown that the lower the income, the smaller the percentage of users. This effect of income was weaker in the free health care (0% user charge rate) group and increased with higher user charge rates. These results supported the hypothesis that a high user charge rate causes people to refrain from receiving health care, and that this effect is stronger in people with lower income.

Table 4.1: Results of logistic regression analysis of the probability that the consumption of prescription drugs would be reduced if the user charge (co-payment) increased

Explanatory variable	B-estimate	S.E.	Significance level (two sided P-values)
Constant	−0.6596	0.4011	0.1000
Percentage user charge increase	0.0105	0.0012	<0.0001
Gender[a]	−0.1725	0.1516	0.2552
Age			
30–39[b]	0.1485	0.2026	0.4635
40–49[b]	−0.1388	0.2212	0.5304
50–59[b]	−0.3394	0.2566	0.1859
60–69[b]	−0.2733	0.2789	0.3272
70–79[b]	−1.1928	0.3158	0.0002
80–84[b]	−0.7143	0.4311	0.0975
10–14 999 SEK[c]	−0.5372	0.1557	0.0006
15–19 999 SEK[c]	−0.3798	0.2055	0.0646
>20 000 SEK[c]	−1.1938	0.3248	0.0002
High school[d]	−0.2498	0.1688	0.1387
University[d]	−0.5734	0.1957	0.0034
Unemployed	0.4882	0.2978	0.1011
Fair health[d]	−0.4688	0.3414	0.1697
Good health[d]	−0.6911	0.3370	0.0403
Very good health[d]	−1.1615	0.3364	0.0011
Excellent health[d]	−0.7711	0.3760	0.0403
Medication			
Penicillin	0.0734	0.2416	0.7324
Analgesics	−0.9910	0.1844	0.5909
Skin creams	0.1068	0.2042	0.6011
Vitamin preparations	−0.1250	0.2567	0.6262
Gastric drugs	−0.1874	0.2779	0.5003
Antidepressants	−0.2719	0.3761	0.4697
Gastric ulcer drugs	−0.3268	0.3958	0.4089
Sedatives	0.2948	0.2948	0.3174
Cardiac drugs	−0.2907	0.3670	0.4284
Hypnotics	−0.1935	0.3108	0.5335
Antiallergics	0.3124	0.3094	0.3126
Antianginal	−0.4081	0.4806	0.3957
Contraceptives	0.3048	0.2093	0.1453

Table 4.1: continued

Antidiarrheal/constipation	0.5215	0.3114	0.0940
Antihypertensives	−0.4255	0.2158	0.0486
Climacteric drugs	−0.7009	0.3067	0.0223
Antitussives	0.9861	0.2464	0.0001
Number of observations	2008		
Log-likelihood value	−832.75		
Goodness of fit	2,040.98		
Likelihood ration index	0.11		
Individual prediction (%)	82.27		

Notes.
a: Coded as 0 = man, 1 = woman.
b: Baseline category is 20–29 years.
c: Baseline category is <999 SEK.
d: Baseline category is less than high school.
e: Baseline category is poor health.

The percentage of participants who accessed in-patient care was higher in the low income bracket. This is because the upper limits of user charges were set according to income. This made it more likely for those in the low income bracket to have user charges in excess of the upper limit imposed if they received in-patient care, which tends to be expensive.

In the individual deductible subgroup, the user charge rate was as high as 95%. It was expected that the participants in this subgroup would refrain from receiving out-patient care, which tends to be inexpensive. They were also expected to not hesitate in receiving expensive care whose cost would exceed the upper limit of user charges. The percentage of those who received any health care in this subgroup was comparable to that in the 50% user charge rate group. On the other hand, the percentage of participants in this subgroup who accessed in-patient care was higher than in the 25% group. The individual deductible subgroup had easier access to expensive in-patient care because the upper limit of user charges was set at $150 regardless of income. These results seem to reflect the fact that the individual deductible subgroup had no advantage in inexpensive health care, whose cost would not exceed the upper limit, and that those with higher income had easier access to this kind of health care. It seems that setting upper limits of user charges according to

Table 4.2: Annual use of medical services per capita by plan (standard errors in parentheses)[a]

	Likelihood of any use (%)	Outpatient expenditures (1991 $)	Face-to-face visits	One or more admissions (%)	Total expenditures (1991 $)	Total admissions	Inpatient expenditure (1991 $)	Number of person-years
Plan								
Free	86.8 (0.8)	446 (14)	4.55 (0.17)	10.3 (0.45)	982 (50.7)	0.128 (0.0070)	536 (42)	6,822
25%	78.7 (1.4)	341 (20)	3.33 (0.19)	8.4 (0.61)	831 (69.2)	0.105 (0.0070)	489 (56)	4,065
50%	77.2 (2.3)	294 (22)	3.03 (0.22)	7.2 (0.77)	884 (189.1)	0.092 (0.0166)	590 (182)	1,401
95%	67.7 (1.8)	266 (16)	2.73 (0.18)	7.9 (0.55)	679 (58.7)	0.099 (0.0078)	413 (49)	3,727
Individual deductible	72.3 (1.5)	308 (16)	3.02 (0.17)	9.6 (0.55)	797 (60.3)	0.115 (0.0076)	489 (55)	4,175
$\chi^2(4)$[b]	144.7	85.3	68.8	19.5	15.9	11.7	4.1	
p-value for χ^2	2.8×10^{-30}	1.3×10^{-17}	4.1×10^{-14}	0.0006	0.003	0.02	Not significant	
p-value for free vs. 95% contrast[c]	1.6×10^{-22}	2.0×10^{-17}	1.0×10^{-13}	0.00037	0.000051	0.0028	0.027	
Noise index	0.009	0.0032	0.037	0.044	0.052	0.055	0.078	

Notes.

a: The values in the table are sample means by plan. All standard errors are corrected for intertemporal and intrafamily correlation using an approach due to Huber; see text. Dollars are expressed in 1991 dollars. Visits are face-to-face contacts with M.D., D.O., or other health providers and exclude visits for only radiology, anaesthesiology, or pathology services. All data exclude dental services and outpatient psychotherapy services. The sample includes children born into the study except for the year of birth and excludes partial years except for deaths.

b: Testing null hypothesis of no difference among plans.

c: p-value comes from 1-tail t-test.

d: Value shown is coefficient of variation in free-care plan.

income will curb access to out-patient care and control access to more important in-patient care.

One of the goals to be achieved by increasing user charge rates was to reduce inappropriate health care. In order to find out whether this goal was achieved, the study analysed the appropriateness of in-patient care provided (Table 4.3). Two physicians reviewed relevant medical records based on common criteria for assessment and examined whether the provision of in-patient care was appropriate. For the purposes of this examination, cases of in-patient care with no medical advantage for patients were regarded as 'inappropriate admissions'. A certain day within each period of in-patient care was selected and assessed as to the appropriateness of the care provided on that day.

The proportion of inappropriate admissions did not differ between the participants who had user charges imposed and those who were entitled to free health care. It was shown that access to in-patient care was curbed regardless of whether the care was appropriate or inappropriate. The results did not support the expectation that appropriate care would not be curbed very much by the imposition of user charges; nor did they provide evidence that user charges curb inappropriate health care only. Similarly, no difference was observed in the proportion of inappropriate admission. It seems that the choice of health care service provided does not depend on whether user charges are imposed. An analysis of the degree of severity also showed no difference between those who had access to free health care and those who were paying user charges. It was not observed that participants who were entitled to free health care tended to consult before symptoms appeared or became serious, or that those for whom high user charges were imposed tended to seek access to health care later and consult after symptoms had become more severe.

The Rand Health Insurance Experiment showed that the higher the user charge rate, the more strongly health care access was curbed, and that this effect was stronger in lower income earners. Health care access also depended on the upper limit of income or user charges. However, the imposition of user charges curbed not only unnecessary health care but also necessary health care. In addition, it was not observed that the imposition of user charges delayed participants' access to in-patient care or caused an increase in the degree of disease severity.

The results of the Rand Health Insurance Experiment mentioned in this chapter represent only some of the study's overall results.

Table 4.3: Rates of adult medical-surgical hospitalisations by insurance plans[a]

	Free plan	Cost sharing for all services	Individual deductible
Enrolees (no.)	1,098	1,535	780
Admissions (no.)	486	504	278
Response rate (%)[b]	90.5	88.5	88.5
Total medical-surgical admissions[c]	126 ± 19	96 ± 13[d]	109 ± 20
Appropriate admissions[c]	96 ± 15	75 ± 11[d]	82 ± 17
Inappropriate admissions[c]	30 ± 15	22 ± 5[e]	26 ± 9
Total hospital days[c]	830 ± 159	640 ± 110	842 ± 241
Inappropriate days[c]	292 ± 83	213 ± 53[f]	324 ± 107
Inappropriate admissions[c] (%)	24 ± 4	22 ± 4[f]	24 ± 7
Inappropriate days[c] (%)	35 ± 6	34 ± 6[f]	38 ± 10
Inappropriate days[c] per admission (%)	2.3 ± 0.6	2.2 ± 0.5[f]	3.0 ± 0.8

Notes.
a: 95% confidence intervals are presented for al plans.
b: Percent of admissions.
c: Per 1,000 person-years.
d: p 0.0.5 vs. free plan.
e: The significance of this difference between the free and cost sharing plans is sensitive to the method of analysis used. If only simple means are analysed, $p = 0.06$; however $p = 0.015$ when a multiple regression model is used.
f: The significance of the difference between the free and cost-sharing plans is sensitive to the method of analysis used. If only simple means are analysed, $p = 0.11$; however, $p = 0.02$ when a multiple regression model is used.

Analyses have been made from several aspects, including the upper limits of user charges or income, gender and age, and emergency or preventive care. The Rand Health Insurance Experiment is a valuable study to this day as a comprehensive intervention study which showed the effect of user charges in the setting of health insurance.

AIDS patients and anti-HIV combination therapy

AIDS has become a social problem in Thailand. According to estimates, as of the year 2000, 700,000 people have been infected with

HIV, 55,000 people have developed AIDS, and the HIV prevalence rates are 2% and 1% in adult men and women, respectively. Anti-HIV combination therapies that delay the onset of AIDS are effective but extremely expensive. Only the wealthy classes can afford these therapies at their own expense. Thailand established universal insurance coverage in October 2001. There are three health insurance schemes: the Civil Servant Medical Benefit Scheme (CSMBS), the Social Security Scheme (SSS), and the Universal Coverage Scheme (USC) or 30 Baht Scheme. The different schemes have different health insurance coverage. When the investigation described below was conducted in 2002, anti-HIV combination therapy was covered only by the CSMBS and only if given in in-patient settings. It was thus expected that access to anti-HIV combination therapy was influenced by socioeconomic factors in Thailand.

Under these circumstances, Kitajima and his colleagues conducted an investigation of 361 patients (193 men and 168 women; average age 33.6 ± 6.8 years) with HIV/AIDS who received care at certain hospitals in Khon Kaen Province in the northeast of Thailand[12]. Data collected included HIV stages, treatment received (including laboratory tests and drugs), cost, health care insurance and user charges. The numbers of patients covered by the CSMBS, SSS and UCS were 26 (7.2%), 39 (10.8%) and 217 (60.1%), respectively, while the self-paying patients numbered 79 (21.1%). The patients receiving anti-HIV combination therapy numbered 76, which accounted for 21.1% of all subjects. Of these patients, the CSMBS covered 65%, SS covered 31%, UCS covered 17% and 14% received treatment at their own expense.

After the adjustment of the patients' background data using logistical regression analysis, it was revealed that the CSMBS and the development of AIDS-related diseases were the factors associated with anti-HIV combination therapy. It was shown that the difference in coverage among the different insurance schemes affected AIDS patients' health care access (Table 4.4). The type of insurance reflected social disparities, such as a person's occupation. These social disparities led to the restriction of access to reliable treatment and were strongly related to survival. Currently, certain (mainly developing) countries in which AIDS has become a serious problem are allowed to ignore patents to HIV drugs as an exceptional measure. The Thai government promotes the production of cheap anti-HIV drugs as well as the improvement

Table 4.4: Factors associated with anti-HIV combination therapy (logistic regression analysis)

	Coefficient	(SE)	p value
Being male (vs female)	0.52	(0.30)	0.08
Age (vs 40 years old and above)			
20–29 years old	–0.67	(0.44)	0.13
30–39 years old	–0.43	(0.36)	0.23
Type of insurance (vs UC)			
CSMBS	2.04	(0.48)	<0.01
SS	0.68	(0.41)	0.10
Self-paying	–0.32	(0.39)	0.41
Stage (vs AIDS)			
Asymptomatic	–0.21	(0.50)	0.67
AIDS-related complex	1.07	(0.32)	< 0.01

Source: Kitajima, et al. (2003)[12].

of the universal insurance coverage, in an attempt to improve AIDS patients' access to anti-HIV combination therapy.

Conclusion: health care access and equity

Access to health care is a right of all people and should not be affected by income or wealth[13]. In order to achieve equity of access to health care, health care resources must be distributed fairly and appropriately. Achievement of fair health care is of high ethical value in that it will reduce disparities in health across communities among which social disparities exist[14]. In other words, improvement of access to health care is a key factor for connecting the value of equity to reality. It is also said to be an important indicator for measuring equity[15]. As described in this chapter, improving access to cost-effective preventive measures and promoting equity of access to health care are likely to serve to get rid of inequity in health.

An equality-oriented approach that says all people should receive the same level of health care will probably not be accepted in its entirety. If equity of access were based on the independence of individuals and freedom of choice, it would not necessarily be unfair to expect affluent people to pay for 'additional' health care in their attainment of health care access. One future task in achieving fair health care access is to distribute health care resources in a manner that will meet the various needs of community members.

Different communities have different health issues. Even if the same health issue is shared by different communities, they have different health care needs. Different communities also have different values and priorities. Communities with different needs seek health care access based on different values. It is a more difficult task to proceed from 'horizontal equity', in which all people are entitled to the same health care, to 'vertical equity', in which people are entitled to equivalent health care based on their own values. There has not even been a proposal of a clear guiding principle to assess this vertical equity.

The goal of standardising equal access is not compatible with the development of service, which is based on local needs and priorities. This results in the pursuit of diversity in access. In promoting vertical equity, it is important not to confuse this diversity in access with unfair distribution of resources. A key to future health care planning is to appropriately control the use of health care while maintaining the availability of health care access. To do so, it is important to set specific goals to win the understanding of people with different goals, while maintaining the equity of results of health care.

It is difficult to assess the degree of achievement of equity obtained through improvement of health care access. However, one essential endpoint is the degree of improvement of health care access for the poor and others whose health care access is hindered by social disparities.

Literature

1 Gulliford, M. and M. Morgan (2003), *Access to Health Care*, London: Routledge.
2 Wang, F. and W. Luo (2005), 'Assessing spatial and nonspatial factors for healthcare access: towards an integrated approach to defining health professional shortage areas', *Health and Place*, 11, pp. 131–146.
3 Senior, M., H. Williams and G. Higgs (2000), 'Urban-rural mortality differentials: controlling for material deprivation', *Social Science and Medicine*, 51, pp. 289–305.
4 Hart, J. T. (1971), 'The inverse care law', *Lancet*, 1, pp. 405–412.
5 Leese, B. and N. Bosanquet (1995), 'Change in general practice and its effects on service provision in areas with different socioeconomic characteristics', *British Medical Journal*, 311, pp. 546–550.

6 Baker, D. and E. Middleton (2003), 'Cervical screening and health inequality in England in the 1990s', *Journal of Epidemiology and Community Health*, 57, pp. 417–423.

7 Department of Health (2000), *The NHS plan: a plan for investment: a plan for reform,* London: The Stationery Office (CM 4818–1).

8 Yamaoka, K. and Y. Kobayashi (1994), *Kōdō keiryō gaku shirīzu 4: iryō to shakai no keiryō gaku* (Behaviormetrics series 4: metrics in health care and society), p. 128, Tokyo: Asakura Shoten.

9 Wagstaff, A., E. van Doorslaer and P. Paci (1991), 'On the measurement of horizontal inequity in the delivery of health care', *Journal of Health Economics*, 10, pp. 169–205.

10 Lundberg, L., M. Johannesson, D. G. L. Isacson and L. Borgquist (1998), 'Effects of user charges on the use of prescription medicines in different socio-economic groups', *Health Policy*, 44, pp. 123–134.

11 Newhouse, J. P. and the Insurance Experiment Group (1993), *Free for all? Lessons from the RAND health insurance experiment*, Boston: Harvard University Press.

12 Kitajima, T., Y. Kobayashi, W. Chaipah, H. Sato, W. Chadbunchachai and R. Thuennadee (2003), 'Costs of medical services for patients with HIV/AIDS in Khon Kaen, Thailand', *AIDS*, 17, pp. 2375–2381.

13 Williams, A. (1993), 'Equity in health care: the role of ideology', in E. van Doorslaer, A. Wagstaff and F. Rutten (eds), *Equity in the Finance and Delivery of Health Care: an International Perspective*, pp. 287–298, Oxford: Oxford Medical Publications.

14 Braveman, P., B. Starfield and H. J. Geiger (2001), World Health Report 2000: how it removes equity from the agenda for public health monitoring and policy, *British Medical Journal*, 323, pp. 678–681.

15 Culyer, A. J. and A. Wagstaff (1993), 'Equity and equality in health care', *Journal of Health Economics*, 12, pp. 431–457.

5 Health and Occupational Class
Akizumi Tsutsumi

Health disparities among occupational classes, and job stress

Occupational class and health issues

Along with income and education, occupational class is a typical indicator of socioeconomic status. As with low income and limited education, it has been shown that various health issues are found in higher proportions among workers in lower occupational classes. Health disparities among occupational classes have been observed constantly since the Industrial Revolution. These disparities have been widening in recent years and have attracted the attention of researchers[1-4].

In adult men in England and Wales, the standardised mortality ratios (SMRs) for 1991–1993 were 66 and 189 for professional workers and unskilled workers, respectively, showing a roughly three-fold difference. The SMRs for skilled workers and semi-skilled workers were 117 and 116, respectively. These data show that the SMRs form a steep gradient according to occupational classes (Figure 5.1)[2]. Meanwhile, the total mortality rate decreased during the two decades from 1970–1972 to 1991–1993. However, the differences in SMR among the different occupational classes increased during the same decades. Similar trends were seen for women[3] and even among white-collar workers with relatively uniform jobs[5]. In a twenty-five year follow-up study of approximately 18,000 male civil servants working for the British government, the men in the lowest occupational group were about three times as likely to die between the age of 40 and the pre-retirement age of 64 as those in the highest occupational group.

Occupational class and coronary heart disease

Coronary heart disease (CHD) is the leading cause of death in Western countries. As such, the relationship between CHD and occupational classes has been studied most extensively. Once described as the 'pressure working the machine to its maximum capacity...and the indicator of [someone] whose engine is always at full speed ahead'[6], CHD used to be found more often in upper occupational classes, which are characterised by busy settings and heavy responsibilities. However, the frequencies of CHD occurrence and mortality for different occupational classes reversed from the 1940s through to the 1960s. CHD became more common in lower occupational classes than upper ones. The disparities among occupational classes have been widening in recent years due to the decreased CHD mortality rates in high occupational classes (Figure 5.1)[2, 3, 7–9].

One factor which has been shown to explain this phenomenon is the disparity in exposure to hazardous environments among occupational classes[10]. While the development of technology has steadily reduced physical burdens on workers, those in lower occupational classes are still more likely to be exposed to heat, cold, noise, hazardous substances and other physical and chemical dangers. However, a strong association between occupational classes and health issues has been found even among white-collar workers, who are less exposed to hazardous physical and chemical environmental factors[5]. It can be inferred from this that there is a more fundamental cause for the occupational disparities in CHD occurrence.

Workers in lower occupational classes are more likely to develop CHD because they tend to engage in unhealthy personal behaviours, such as smoking and lack of exercise, and to suffer from obesity[11–13]. Smoking rates have decreased more slowly among blue-collar workers than white-collar, and blue-collar workers are employed in workplaces with less severe restrictions on smoking[14]. In addition, biological risk factors for CHD, such as blood pressure and plasma fibrinogen, are distributed unevenly among occupational classes. However, even if adjustments are made for these established risk factors, the disparities in CDH occurrence and prognosis among occupational classes cannot be fully explained[15, 16]. Related to this, the importance of job stress has drawn close attention since it was pointed out that psychosocial characteristics of jobs could explain the CHD disparities among occupational classes[17].

Psychosocial job stress models

In epidemiological studies attempting to reveal the effect of job stress on health, the big challenge has been to measure complicated invisible stress, which is recognised differently by different

Figure 5.1 SMRs, by social class (based on occupation), males, England and Wales, 1970–72, 1979–80, 82–83, and 1991–93

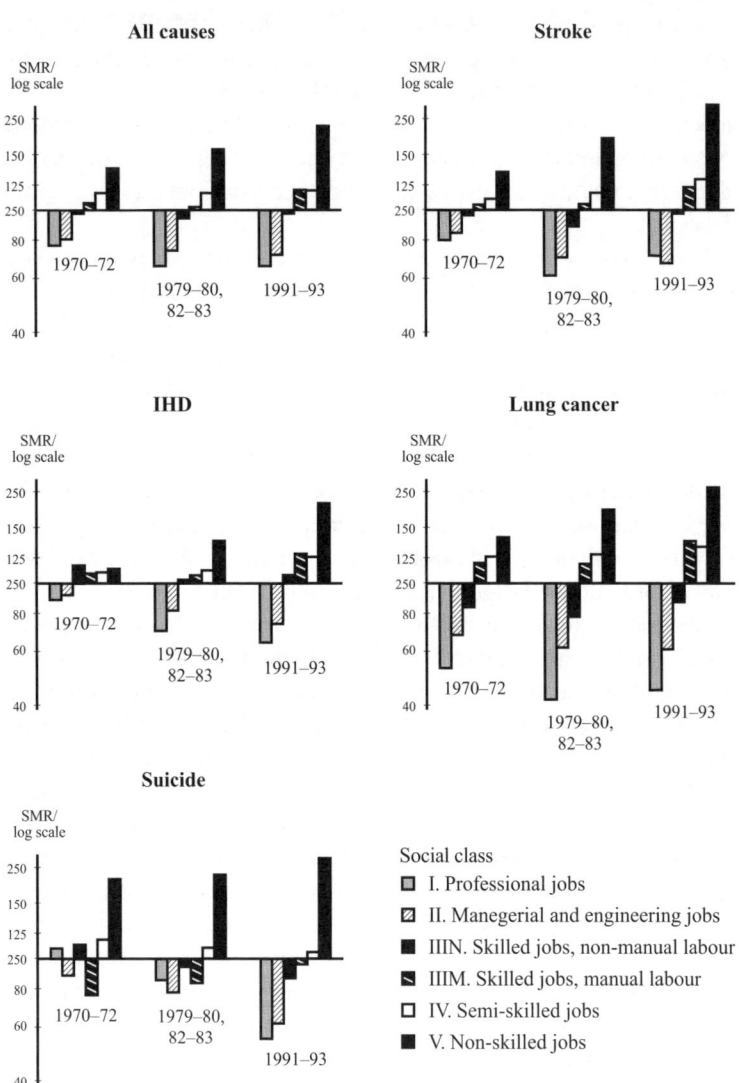

Source: Figure 3 from Drever, Whitehead & Roden (1996)[2]. Reproduced with permission from HMSO.

Figure 5.2: Job demand–control model

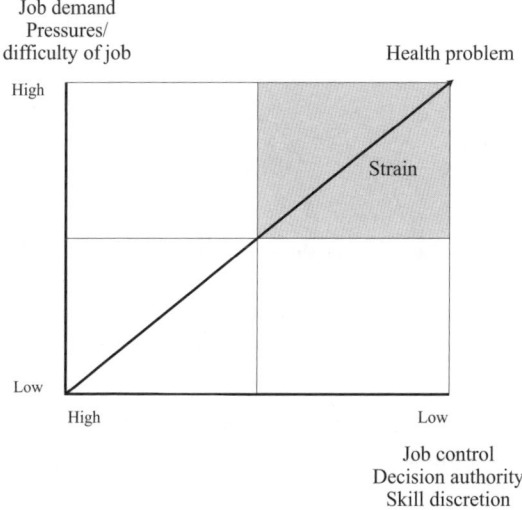

The higher the job demand (speed and workload) and the lower the control (the level of decision authority and skill discretion), the higher the risk of health problems.

individuals. Knowledge of job stress increased dramatically with the adoption of models which assess stress as combinations of characteristics of hazardous jobs. These characteristics have clearly defined concepts and are commonly found in many types of jobs. The job stress models which currently attract most attention are the 'job demand–control' model and the 'effort–reward imbalance' model (Figures 5.2 and 5.3)[18].

Job demand–control model

The job demand–control model consists of two factors: demand and control. Demand is represented by the workload pressure and the psychological pressure of a job. Control is represented by the degree to which one has decision-making authority over the job and the degree to which one uses his/her skills in the job. Workers with high-demand but low-control jobs are exposed to strain and are supposed to have a higher risk of disease.

It has been shown that the demand–control model can predict CHD and various other health problems. Recent studies have shown that a lack of job control has a particularly significant impact on health[19]. It is fair to say that this model has shown not only

Figure 5.3: Effort–reward imbalance model

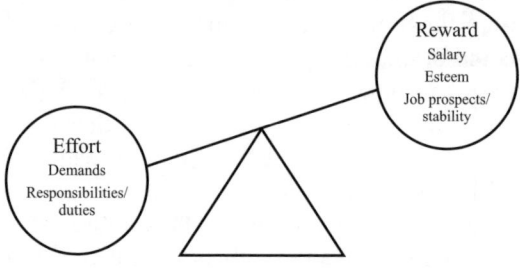

The imbalance between the effort made at work and the reward which should be (or is expected to be) obtained from that work is deemed stressful.

the pressure aspect of jobs, such as a huge workload and heavy responsibility, but also the importance of resources to cope with this aspect of jobs.

Effort–reward imbalance model
The effort–reward imbalance model focuses not only on salary but other reward factors, including esteem, employment stability and prospects. In this model, a working environment is found to be stressful if the effort made in the job is not rewarded with fitting compensation. A large number of studies have demonstrated the hypothesis that various health problems may occur if one is constantly placed in a situation where his/her 'hard work is not recognised/rewarded'[20]. Intensifying international competition and an economic recession in Japan have prompted the restructuring and downsizing of companies, resulting in unstable employment and an increased number of non-regular workers. In the current working environment, the economic and industrial structures are undergoing significant changes. In this work environment, the effort–reward imbalance model has the potential to sensitively measure the stress of workers beyond the level of individual workers' jobs.

Psychosocial job stress and health disparities among occupations

Two hypotheses have been proposed for mechanisms by which job stress explains health disparities among different occupational classes[21, 22]. The uneven distribution of stressors among occupational classes may explain the uneven distribution of health problems.

This is known as the 'mediation mechanism'. With this, workers in lower occupational classes are more exposed to psychosocial job stress than those in upper occupational classes. Although quantitative and/or qualitative workloads are not always heavier in lower classes, the higher one's position is, the higher the reward and the availability of control, support and other resources[23,24]. Also, among blue-collar workers, for whom exposure to physical and chemical stressors has been an issue, it has been shown that control over their own jobs and prospects is limited at a personal level[25]. It has been found that the statistical adjustment of workers' control over their jobs significantly reduces the relative risk of CHD occurrence among workers in lower occupational classes as compared to those in higher occupational classes[26,27].

It has also been observed that the effect of job stress on health is greater in lower than higher occupational classes or, alternatively, that a significant effect on health from stress is found only in lower occupational classes[21,28–32]. The effect explained by the interaction between low occupational class and job stress is known as the 'modification effect'[22].

Empirical studies

This author's group has analysed the mechanisms by which job stress links occupational classes and health problems. Using data on Japanese workers, we analysed (i) whether the stressors defined by the demand–control model and the effort–reward imbalance model are unevenly distributed between different occupational classes and, thus, whether adjustment of this distribution would reduce the health disparities between the occupational classes (the mediation mechanism); or (ii) if the effect of stress on health is stronger in lower occupational classes (the modification effect).

Job demand–control model

Let me first describe findings relating to the job demand–control model. People who received a general health check-up under the Health and Medical Service Law for the Aged during the period 1992–1995 were invited to participate in the Jichi Medical School (JMS) cohort study. 4,911 men and 7,579 women from twelve municipalities participated in the study[33]. Of these participants, those who were employed at a baseline level were questioned about certain items relating to their work environments. This population is characterised by a high proportion of workers in primary industries, unlike previous studies on job stress and health issues whose subjects were workers employed by relatively large companies. The JMS cohort study used the demand–control model questionnaires used in the MONICA study. The coefficients of reliability for the job demand scale (five items) and the job control scale (six items) were 0.70 and 0.64, respectively. The ratio of the score on the demand scale to that on the control scale was used as an indicator of strain.

Demand–control model stress indicators among occupations
The distribution of scores on the demand and control scales was compared by gender among different occupational classes. With the exception of the demand scores between female white- and blue-collar workers, workers in the upper occupational classes had higher demand scores and control scores than those in their corresponding lower occupational classes. Strain levels were significantly higher for workers in lower positions and among blue-collar workers (Table 5.1)[34]. These results mean that job demand is not necessarily higher, but that job control is lower in the groups representing lower occupational classes than those representing higher occupational classes. This shows, as expected, uneven distribution of strain as a composite indicator of job demand and control among the occupational classes.

Next, let me describe our attempt to explain the relationship between occupational class and coronary risk factors by the job demand–control model using plasma fibrinogen levels and the prevalence of hypertension as outcomes.

Analysis using plasma fibrinogen levels
An elevated plasma fibrinogen level is a coronary risk factor. Plasma fibrinogen levels are associated not only with age, heredity and other biological factors but also with socioeconomic factors and health behaviour. Some of the municipalities that participated in the JMS cohort study measured plasma fibrinogen levels of their subjects, and we analysed these subjects: 1,794 male and 1,942 female workers[35].

First, we analysed whether there was any disparity in plasma fibrinogen levels among the occupational classes and whether the disparity, if any, would be reduced by adjusting the indicator of job stress (strain) (Table 5.2).

Table 5.1: *Comparison of stress levels between occupational classes based on demand–control model (JMS cohort study; baseline, 1992/1995)*

	Male				Female			
	n	Demand	Control	Strain[a]	n	Demand	Control	Strain
All subjects	3187	11.9	16.9	0.718	3400	10.8	14.9	0.753
Position								
Administrators/ managers	1595	12.3[c]	17.5[c]	0.711[c]	945	11.1[c]	15.4[c]	0.744[c]
General workers	1290	11.5	16.1	0.736	2029	10.7	14.5	0.768
Occupational category								
White-collar	893	12.1[b]	17.4[c]	0.705[b]	1429	10.6[b]	15.3[c]	0.718[c]
Blue-collar	2241	11.8	16.7	0.724	1931	10.9	14.7	0.778

Notes.
a: Strain, demand score/control score.
b: $p < 0.01$
c: $p < 0.001$.
Source: modified from Tsutsumi, et al. (2001)[34].

The male blue-collar workers had higher fibrinogen levels than their white-collar counterparts. This relationship was somewhat reduced by adjusting fibrinogen-related factors but remained statistically significant. Adjustment of strain did not reduce the remarkable association. No considerable difference was observed in plasma fibrinogen levels between administrators/managers and general workers. Despite there being a large number of older, postmenopausal workers, female administrators and managers had significantly lower plasma fibrinogen levels than other female workers. This association was not explained by adjusting potential confounding factors, including strain.

These results show that in this cohort, while some gender differences were seen due to the manner of classification of occupational classes, there were disparities in plasma fibrinogen levels between the corresponding occupational classes, and these disparities were not affected significantly by adjusting the stress indicator.

Table 5.2: Relation between occupational classes and plasma fibrinogen levels – results of multivariate linear regression analysis (JMS cohort study, 1992/1995)

	Male (n = 1794)					Female (n = 1942)				
	B	SE	β	t	p	B	SE	β	t	p
Administrators/managers vs. other [a]										
Model I [b]	2.292	2.616	0.021	0.876	0.381	6.836	2.537	0.061	2.695	0.007
Model II [c]	1.771	2.494	0.017	0.710	0.478	6.150	2.573	0.055	2.390	0.017
Model III [d]	1.013	2.506	0.010	0.404	0.686	6.594	2.641	0.059	2.496	0.013
White-collar vs. blue-collar [e]										
Model I	9.616	2.801	0.081	3.433	0.001	−4.475	2.388	−0.044	−1.914	0.056
Model II	7.230	2.690	0.064	2.698	0.007	−4.155	2.348	−0.041	−1.769	0.077
Model III	6.744	2.691	0.060	2.507	0.012	−4.559	2.451	−0.045	−1.860	0.063

Notes.
a: Administrators/managers, 0; other, 1.
b: Model I, adjusted for age.
c: Model II, adjusted for age, smoking, alcohol consumption, BMI and total cholesterol.
d: Model III, adjusted for age, smoking, alcohol consumption, BMI, total cholesterol and strain.
e: White-collar, 0; blue-collar, 1.
Source: Tsutsumi, et al. (1998)[35].

Next, we analysed whether or not the degree of association between strain and plasma fibrinogen levels was different between the corresponding occupational classes (Table 5.3). For male workers, strain was significantly related to plasma fibrinogen levels (B = 3.038, SE = 1.523, β = 0.048, t = 2.024, p = 0.043). This relationship was stronger in blue-collar workers than white-collar. No difference was observed between administrators/managers and general workers. For female workers, strain had a negative association with plasma fibrinogen levels in white-collar workers and administrators/managers, although statistical significance was not reached. Among female blue-collar workers and general workers, strain had a positive association with plasma fibrinogen levels. These results suggest that the relationship between strain and plasma fibrinogen levels was stronger in lower occupational groups (the modification effect).

Table 5.3: Relation between strain[a] and plasma fibrinogen by occupational class – results of multivariate linear regression analysis [b] (JMS cohort study, 1992/1995)

	Male (n = 1794)					Female (n = 1942)				
	B	SE	β	t	p	B	SE	β	t	p
Position										
Administrators/ managers	3.110	2.151	0.049	1.446	0.149	–3.557	2.654	–0.059	–1.340	0.181
Other	3.078	2.169	0.047	1.419	0.156	2.244	1.699	0.036	1.321	0.187
Occupational category										
White-collar workers	0.221	2.426	0.004	0.091	0.927	–0.080	2.066	–0.001	–0.039	0.969
Blue-collar workers	3.789	1.905	0.056	1.989	0.047	2.901	1.984	0.047	1.462	0.144

Notes.
a: The distribution of the ratio of demand scores to control scores was divided into three categories for each gender. The categories were coded 1, 2 and 3 in ascending order of presumed strain levels and were put into the model.
b: Adjusted for gender, smoking, alcohol consumption, BMI and total cholesterol.

Analysis using prevalence of hypertension

We analysed 3,187 male and 3,400 female workers under sixty-five years of age who had no missing values in their blood pressure data and demand–control questionnaires, using the prevalence of hypertension as the outcome[34]. Workers whose systolic blood pressure was over 160 mmHg or diastolic blood pressure was over 90 mmHg, or who had been diagnosed with hypertension by physicians were defined as hypertensive. The systolic and diastolic blood pressures were measured with a fully automated sphygmomanometer after each subject had been sitting for five minutes.

The age-adjusted prevalence of hypertension tended to be higher in the upper occupational classes in both genders. No disparity in the prevalence of hypertension was seen between the corresponding occupational classes. Adjustment for strain did not affect the relationship between occupational classes and the prevalence of hypertension.

However, a significant association was observed between strain and the prevalence of hypertension in male workers. Among all occupational groups, the high strain groups tended to have higher prevalence of hypertension, although the risk reached statistical significance only in the lower occupational classes (the risk of hypertension increased in relation to strain among administrators/managers and other workers: adjusted odds ratio [AOR], 1.08; 95% confidence interval [CI], 0.92–1.27 and AOR, 1.31; 95% CI, 1.09–1.58, respectively, and in white-collar and blue-collar workers, AOR, 1.11; 95% CI, 0.90–1.37 and AOR, 1.20; 95% CI, 1.05–1.38, respectively). In female workers, no significant association was observed between strain and the prevalence of hypertension.

These results suggest that in male workers, the effect of job strain on the prevalence of hypertension was stronger in the lower occupational classes (the modification effect).

Effort–reward imbalance model

Effort–reward imbalance model stress indicators among occupations

We attempted to compare the distribution of stress indicators used in the effort–reward imbalance model among different occupational categories, classified according to the International Standard Classification of Occupations (ISCO–88)[36]. The subjects were 21,967 regular workers under sixty years of age employed at thirty-four workplaces all over Japan[37].

We employed the globally-used effort scale (with six items) and reward scale (eleven items)[24]. Both scales were scored with a five-point gradation. Higher total scores on the items meant higher stresses and strains from the occupational environment. The effort–reward score ratios were calculated by dividing effort item scores by reward item scores converted onto a reversed point scale (higher scores meant higher reward), followed by multiplication by a factor correcting the difference in the number of items.

Table 5.4 shows the frequencies of an effort–reward imbalance and of a stressed condition on the effort scores and the reward scores (in each case, the top tertile in the distribution by gender was defined as exposed), expressed as age-adjusted odds ratios against managerial workers.

Among male workers, the frequency of effort–reward imbalance was higher for professionals and technicians, service/sales workers, and plant workers/machine operators, and lower among skilled workers than managers. These trends reached statistical significance. When analysed by categorising the occupations as white-collar or blue-collar, the frequency of effort–reward imbalance was higher for white-collar workers than blue-collar. Effort scores were significantly higher among professionals and service/sales workers than for managers. Technicians, clerical workers, skilled workers, plant workers/machine operators and manual workers had significantly lower effort scores. In the analysis of white-collar versus blue-collar workers, the latter had significantly lower effort scores. On the other hand, reward scores indicated that for all occupations (except skilled workers) there were higher stress levels than for managers.

Among female workers, the frequency of effort–reward imbalance was higher for professionals and lower among clerical and manual workers. The effort level was highest for professionals and was significantly lower for technicians, clerical workers, service/sales workers, plant workers/machine operators and manual workers. The analysis of white-collar versus blue-collar workers showed that managers had the highest effort level. On the other hand, the reward scores indicated that managers had the lowest stress levels, with the difference from other workers reaching statistical significance, except for manual workers.

Next, we compared the stress indices between regular (full-time) and non-regular (part-time) workers (Table 5.5). The effort–reward imbalance level was significantly higher among 'temps' (or 'dispatched workers') than regular workers. For both genders, the reward levels were remarkably different (higher stress for 'temps'). On the other hand, male part-time workers had a lower stress level on the effort scale, and a higher stress level on the reward scale than regular workers. Female part-time workers had lower scores than regular workers on both effort and reward scales and had a lower stress level in the effort–reward imbalance, which reached statistical significance.

The stress levels shown by the effort–reward imbalance model suggest that stress levels are not always higher in lower occupational classes. However, despite the small number of subjects, dispatched workers showed significantly higher stress levels than regular workers for both genders.

Analysis using depression as outcome

Unfortunately, there have only been a small number of studies in Japan that have analysed the effect of the effort–reward imbalance model indicators on CHD and its risk factors. We have used depressive symptoms, which have been presumed to have a causal relationship with the development of CHD[19], as an alternative outcome, and have analysed whether the stress indicators used in

Table 5.4: Relationships between occupational classes and effort–reward stress indicators: age-adjusted odds ratios (OR) and 95% confidence intervals (95% CI) in regular workers under 60 years of age

	n	Effort–reward imbalance [a]			Effort score indicator [b]			Reward score indicator [c]		
		n (%)	OR	95% CI	n (%)	OR	95% CI	n (%)	OR	95% CI
Male										
Professionals	364–376	160 (44.0)	2.18	1.73–2.76	214 (56.9)	1.74	1.38–2.18	125 (34.2)	1.64	1.29–2.08
Technicians	2,840–2,953	1,036 (36.5)	1.33	1.17–1.50	1,219 (41.3)	0.85	0.75–0.95	1,157 (40.4)	1.79	1.59–2.02
Clerks	1,837–1,933	557 (30.3)	1.01	0.88–1.16	690 (35.7)	0.69	0.61–0.79	602 (32.3)	1.23	1.08–1.41
Sevice/sales workers	760–795	345 (45.4)	1.98	1.67–2.36	449 (56.5)	1.61	1.36–1.90	316 (41.1)	1.89	1.59–2.24
Skilled workers	1,098–1,140	218 (19.9)	0.67	0.56–0.81	340 (29.8)	0.53	0.45–0.63	254 (22.8)	0.94	0.79–1.11
Plant and machine operators	1,932–2,040	740 (38.3)	1.55	1.36–1.76	747 (36.6)	0.82	0.73–0.93	870 (43.9)	2.04	1.80–2.31
Manual workers	774–812	227 (29.3)	0.94	0.79–1.12	278 (34.2)	0.70	0.59–0.83	289 (37.0)	1.40	1.18–1.66
Managers	2,745–2,903	838 (30.5)	1.00		1,095 (37.7)	1.00		886 (31.9)	1.00	
White-collar workers	5,801–6,057	2,098 (36.2)	1.36	1.22–1.52	2,572 (42.5)	0.92	0.83–1.02	2,200 (37.5)	1.64	1.48–1.82
Blue-collar workers	3,804–3,992	1,185 (31.2)	1.15	1.03–1.29	1,365 (34.2)	0.71	0.64–0.79	1,413 (36.4)	1.59	1.42–1.77

		Effort–reward imbalance [a]			Effort score indicator [b]			Reward score indicator [c]		
	n	n (%)	OR	95% CI	n (%)	OR	95% CI	n (%)	OR	95% CI
Female										
Professionals	2,199–2,384	977 (44.4)	1.81	1.33–2.47	1,320 (55.4)	1.78	1.34–2.38	678 (30.4)	1.43	1.05–1.95
Technicians	737–802	198 (26.9)	0.73	0.53–1.02	182 (22.7)	0.42	0.31–0.57	320 (42.5)	2.01	1.47–2.75
Clerks	994–1,061	205 (20.6)	0.53	0.38–0.73	171 (16.1)	0.27	0.20–0.37	356 (35.2)	1.52	1.11–2.07
Sevice/sales workers	194–222	55 (28.4)	0.81	0.53–1.24	60 (27.0)	0.53	0.36–0.79	85 (42.5)	2.07	1.39–3.08
Skilled workers	12–18	4 (33.3)	0.95	0.28–3.30	4 (22.2)	0.41	0.13–1.28	8 (61.5)	4.40	1.38–14.07
Plant and machine operators	392–462	146 (37.2)	1.20	0.86–1.68	55 (11.9)	0.21	0.14–0.30	215 (54.3)	3.08	2.20–4.30
Manual workers	168–188	34 (20.2)	0.53	0.34–0.84	28 (14.9)	0.27	0.17–0.44	58 (33.7)	1.35	0.89–2.04
Managers	274–320	85 (31.0)	1.00		117 (36.6)	1.00		78 (28.1)	1.00	
White-collar workers	4,124–4,469	1,435 (34.8)	0.91	0.67–1.21	1,733 (38.8)	0.64	0.48–0.82	1,439 (34.3)	1.65	1.23–2.21
Blue-collar workers	572–668	184 (32.2)	0.89	0.65–1.22	87 (13.0)	0.20	0.14–0.28	281 (48.4)	2.48	1.81–3.39

Notes.

a: The effort scale scores were divided by the reward scale scores converted onto a reversed point scale, followed by multiplication by a factor correcting the difference in the number of items on each scale. For each gender, the top tertile of the distribution of the value so calculated was defined as the exposure standard.

b: For each gender, the top tertile of the distribution of the effort scale scores was defined as the exposure standard.

c: For each gender, the top tertile (high stress) of the distribution of the reward scale scores was defined as the exposure standards.

Source: Tsutsumi & Kawakami (2005)[37].

Table 5.5: Comparison of effort–reward stress indicators between regular and non-regular workers: age-adjusted odds ratios (OR) and 95% confidence intervals (95% CI) in workers under 60 years of age

	n	Effort–reward imbalance[a]			Effort score indicator[b]			Reward score indicator[c]		
		n (%)	OR	95% CI	n (%)	OR	95% CI	n (%)	OR	95% CI
Male										
Regular workers	13,606–14,227	4,528 (33.3)	1.00		5,657 (39.8)	1.00		4,937 (35.8)	1.00	
Dispatched workers	489–505	326 (66.7)	4.68	3.84–5.69	220 (43.6)	1.07	0.89–1.28	416 (84.2)	12.39	9.66–15.89
Part-time workers	95–102	27 (28.4)	1.06	0.67–1.67	26 (25.5)	0.60	0.38–0.94	39 (40.2)	1.63	1.07–2.47
Female										
Regular workers	5,232–5,735	1,761 (33.7)	1.00		1,995 (34.8)	1.00		1,890 (35.5)	1.00	
Dispatched workers	147–164	72 (49.0)	1.85	1.33–2.57	45 (27.4)	0.77	0.54–1.09	107 (71.8)	4.14	2.88–5.95
Part-time workers	2,769–3,447	535 (19.3)	0.51	0.45–0.58	654 (19.0)	0.60	0.53–0.68	755 (26.6)	0.55	0.49–0.62

Notes:

a: The effort scale scores were divided by the reward scale scores converted onto a reversed point scale, followed by multiplication by a factor correcting the difference in the number of items on each scale. For each gender, the top tertile of the distribution of the value so calculated was defined as the exposure standard.

b: For each gender, the top tertile of the distribution of the effort scale scores was defined as the exposure standard.

c: For each gender, the top tertile (high stress) of the distribution of the reward scale scores was defined as the exposure standards.

the effort–reward imbalance model can explain the health disparities among different occupational classes.

We conducted a questionnaire survey which included the effort–reward imbalance model scale and the Center for Epidemiologic Studies Depression Scale (CES-D). The subjects were local public body employees. Of these subjects, 3,856 white-collar workers who were classified as managers, technicians and clerks (based on the ISCO-88) were analysed. For the convenience of data collection, job titles of 'assistant manager' and above were classified as 'managers'.

The prevalence of depressive symptoms was low for managers (the proportion of subjects whose CES-D scores were sixteen points or higher was 15% among managers, while the corresponding proportions for technicians and clerks were 22% and 23%, respectively). The managers were older and included a higher proportion of males, and had a lower education than the technicians and clerks. The proportion of managers who worked over fifty hours per week was low. The proportion of subjects in the top quartile of the distribution of effort–reward imbalance ratio was highest in technicians (32%) and similar in clerks and managers (22% and 23%, respectively). Thus, no trend was observed that indicated higher stress levels in lower occupational classes.

With managers serving as the reference group, we measured the risk of developing depressive symptoms in other occupational categories using odds ratios (OR) adjusted for gender, age, education, working hours and workplace conditions. A trend was observed in that the risk increased among technicians and, to a higher degree, clerks (OR, 1.71; 95% CI, 1.21–2.41 and OR, 1.84; 95% CI, 1.28–2.61, respectively). However, adjustment of the effort–reward imbalance stress indicators reduced the relative risk by only 12% for technicians and had almost no effect among clerks (OR, 1.51; 95% CI, 1.04–2.21 and OR, 1.90; 95% CI, 1.28–2.80, respectively).

Next, we created a cross tabulation based on occupational categories and exposure to stress. With the group of managers without stress exposure serving as the reference group, the risk of developing depression in other groups was measured (Table 5.6). Compared to the group of managers with a good effort–reward balance (low stress), the odds ratio for the group of non-managers with a poor effort–reward balance was equivalent to the product obtained by multiplying the risk involved in being a non-manager by the risk involved in having a poor effort–reward balance.

Table 5.6: Risk of depression calculated for different combinations of effort–reward imbalance and occupational class: odds ratios (OR), 95% confidence intervals (95% CI) and effects of interaction calculated by multivariate logistic analysis (in local public body employees, 2003/2004)

	Administrators		Technicians		AP_{AB}^{a}	S_{AB}^{b}	95% CI^c of S_{AB}
	OR	95% CI	OR	95% CI			
Unadjusted							
Balanced	1.00		1.43	1.06–1.93			
Imbalance	5.18	3.76–7.14	6.61	4.90–8.91	15	1.55	0.84–1.76
Adjusted^c							
Balanced	1.00		1.46	0.86–2.46			
Imbalance	4.56	3.09–6.75	7.43	4.50–12.25	32	1.60	0.77–3.31
	Administrators		Clerical workers		AP_{AB}^{a}	S_{AB}^{b}	95% CI^c of S_{AB}
	OR	95% CI	OR	95% CI			
Unadjusted							
Balanced	1.00		1.91	1.43–2.55			
Imbalance	5.18	3.76–6.91	8.64	6.11–12.23	30	1.50	1.00–2.24
Adjusted^d							
Balanced	1.00		1.81	1.09–3.03			
Imbalance	4.68	3.17–6.91	8.96	5.23–15.34	39	1.77	0.98–3.20

Notes.

a: The percentage of contribution of interaction to depression risk calculated from OR: $AP_{AB} = \dfrac{OR_{AB} - OR_A - OR_B + 1}{OR_{AB}}$

b: Synergy Index: $S_{AB} = \dfrac{(OR_{AB} - 1)}{(OR_A + OR_B) - 2}$ (1 perfectly additive, > 1 synergistic interaction)

[Source: Rothman (1986)[38]]

c: Confidence interval [Source: Hosmer & Lemeshow (1992)[39]]

d: Adjusted for age, gender, education, working hours and workplace.

These analytical results suggest that the adverse effect of effort–reward imbalance is greater in lower than higher occupational classes (the modification effect).

Psychosocial job stress, occupational classes and health

Our analysis showed that in the demand–control model, there was a gradient in the distribution of stress indicators among occupational classes. On the other hand, there was no clear gradient in the distribution of effort–reward imbalance among occupational classes classified according to the ISCO, although it was suggested that the frequency of effort–reward imbalance was higher in dispatched workers than regular workers. In addition, it was shown that the association between stress indicators and health outcomes was stronger in lower occupational groups, and that job stress was involved in a manner that modifies the relationship between occupational classes and health issues.

Disparities in distribution of job stress among occupational classes

It has been shown that in Western countries, job characteristics used as stress indicators in the demand–control model, particularly job control, show up well in occupational classes [17]. Specifically, workers in lower occupational classes have lower job control. A database containing information on large Japanese companies shows disparities in strain level among occupational classes[40]. The JMS cohort study, too, showed that the demand–control model's stress indicators were reflected clearly in occupational classes. Disparities among occupational classes were seen more prominently in relation to job control, showing good consistency with study results obtained in Western countries (The Whitehall II study)[17].

On the other hand, findings on disparities in effort–reward imbalance among occupational classes have not been consistent. The Whitehall II study suggested disparities in effort–reward imbalance among occupational classes[23]. Conversely, the Work, Lipids and Fibrinogen (WOLF) study, which comprised representative samples of Swedish male workers, has shown that higher classes have higher stress levels (Richard Peter, personal communication). However, these two studies used different scales, and further studies are warranted using standardised scales.

In the above-described analysis of data on Japanese workers based on the ISCO, stress levels measured by the effort–reward imbalance model failed to show expected disparities among occupational classes. While the demand–control model attempts to measure stressors arising from jobs, the effort–reward imbalance model attempts to measure those arising from organisational/institutional factors. The database used in the above analysis comprised various occupational categories, including public servants. This makes it likely that the observed association may reflect the influence of the subjects' workplaces, where seniority systems and lifetime employment systems may remain[41]. However, the comparison between dispatched and regular workers showed that the former had significantly higher stress levels. This suggests emerging disparities among occupational classes in Japan, which is experiencing significant changes in employment patterns. In order to confirm the potential uneven distribution of effort–reward imbalance among occupational classes, it is necessary to continue our observation, using more representative samples and paying attention to employment systems.

Mediating effect of job stress

There have often been reports from Western countries that uneven distribution of strain (high demand and low control) among occupational classes explains the disparities in health problems among those classes[26, 27, 42]. In Japan too, Kawakami and his colleagues have shown that most of the linear gradient relationship between occupational class and depression in men can be explained by the difference in job demands and control among occupational categories[43]. In women, these job characteristics explained to some extent the relationship between occupational class and depression, but their effect was minor.

In the JMS cohort study, a disparity in fibrinogen level was seen between white-collar and blue-collar workers among men, and between managers and general workers in women. These trends were not reduced by adjusting for strain. Similar findings have been observed for Japanese male workers employed by large corporations[44]. In addition, our analysis using hypertension as the outcome failed to show expected disparities in the prevalence of hypertension among occupational classes.

The subjects of the JMS cohort study were a relatively old, healthy population[33]. Those who receive medical checkups may be more interested in health than those who do not. In addition, those insured with the Japanese National Health Insurance cannot fully represent a variety of occupations. The subjects' failure to represent the national workforce may be a reason for the failure to confirm the expected disparities in health problems among occupational classes, and for the mediating effect of the demand–control model's stress indicators on the health disparities among occupational classes.

With respect to the effort–reward imbalance model, the WOLF study found higher effort score levels (higher stress) in higher occupational classes, and higher reward score levels (higher stress) in lower occupational classes. In addition, effort scores and reward scores were good predictors of high cholesterol levels in high occupational classes and low occupational classes, respectively. From these results, the researchers who conducted the WOLF study have admitted the possibility that the scales used in the effort–reward imbalance model may mediate the distribution of health problems among occupational classes (Richard Peter, personal communication). However, in our analysis, which used depression in white-collar workers as the outcome, the differences in the frequency of depression among occupational classes were explained only to a small degree by the uneven distribution of effort–reward imbalance among occupational classes.

Modification effect of job stress

With some exceptions[45], it has been frequently observed that the adverse effect of strain on health is greater among workers in lower socioeconomic status occupations[21, 28-32].

In male subjects of the JMS cohort study, the association between strain and plasma fibrinogen levels was stronger in blue-collar workers than white-collar. In female subjects, there was a possibility that the distribution of high plasma fibrinogen levels among occupational classes was modified by strain, but the effect of strain failed to reach statistical significance. Some previous findings may explain the weak association observed among women. For women, it has also been suggested that occupational class has a stronger effect than job stress on plasma fibrinogen levels[46]. In addition, it has been pointed out that the ability of the demand–control model to predict health problems is lower for women than for men[18]. Furthermore, it has been reported that job control, objectively estimated by occupation or position, better predicts plasma fibrinogen levels than self-reported job control[47, 48].

The JMS cohort study showed that again, for male workers, the effect of strain on the prevalence of hypertension was stronger in lower occupational classes. Similar findings have been observed in a study conducted in the West using ambulatory blood pressure as the outcome[49].

Theoretically, the effort–reward imbalance model has a better ability to predict outcomes for workers in lower socioeconomic status jobs, but only a small number of reports have demonstrated this to be true[50]. Our analysis of white-collar workers has shown that the effort–reward imbalance model is likely to predict depressive symptoms for workers in lower occupational classes.

All these studies remain within the bounds of cross-sectional research. Yet our findings suggest that in both the demand–control model and the effort–reward imbalance model, the adverse effects of the stress indicators on health are stronger for workers in lower occupational classes (the modification effect).

Conclusion

In the West, disparities in health problems among various occupational classes have been observed and are increasing. It has been shown that high demand/low control and effort–reward imbalance are good measures of stressors in contemporary occupations, predict various health problems, and explain to a fair degree the disparities in health problems among occupational classes. Although it is difficult to make changes in the existing occupational classes, it is possible to intervene in the area of harmful working environments. This is why it is important to understand the effect of occupational class on health from the viewpoint of job stress. As a health policy measure for workers, active attempts have been made to redesign working environments by manipulating stressors revealed by job stress models[51, 52].

We must wait for further studies before judging whether the relationship between occupational class, CHD and job stress (the last linking the former two) observed in Western countries directly applies to Japan, which has a different working culture and a low incidence of CHD. In Japan, the distribution of coronary risk factors, as well as that of high job stress, does not always show the same trends among occupational classes as those observed in the West[53]. Amid significant changes in working environments, it is imperative to accumulate observation data over time.

The wave of economic globalisation has reached the shores of Japan. While some high-income workers have emerged as a result of the adoption of a merit system, downsizing has resulted in an increase in the number of non-voluntary unemployed. Under these circumstances, various occupational disparities have recently emerged, as seen in the newly-coined Japanese terms, *kachigumi* ('winners') and *makegumi* ('losers'). There has been concern over health issues in non-regular workers[54]. It has also been suggested that the adverse effect of job stress is stronger for workers with unstable employment[55]. As socioeconomic factors having significant effects on the health of workers today, occupational class and job stress seem to be promising areas for intervention measures.

Literature

1 Marmot, M. and T. Theorell (1988), 'Social class and cardiovascular disease: the contribution of work', *International Journal of Health Services*, 18, pp. 659–674.
2 Drever, F., M. Whitehead and M. Roden (1996), 'Current patterns and trends in male mortality by social class (based on occupation)', *Population Trends*, 86, pp. 15–20.
3 Marmot, M. G. and M. E. McDowall (1987), 'Mortality decline and widening social inequalities', *Lancet*, 2, pp. 274–276.
4 Kagamimori, S., Y. Iibuchi and J. Fox (1983), 'A comparison of socio-economic differences in mortality between Japan and England and Wales', *World Health Statistic Quarterly*, 36, pp. 119–128.
5 Marmot, M. G. and M. J. Shipley (1996), 'Do socioeconomic differences in mortality persist after retirement? 25 year follow up of civil servants from the first Whitehall study', *British Medical Journal*, 313, pp. 1177–1180.
6 Osler, W. (1910), The Lumleian Lectures on angina pectoris, *Lancet*, 1, pp. 839–844.
7 Wing, S., E. Barnett, M. Casper and H. A. Tyroler (1992), 'Geographic and socioeconomic variation in the onset of decline of coronary heart disease mortality in white women', *American Journal of Public Health*, 82, pp. 204–209.
8 Marmot, M. G. (1992), 'Coronary heart disease: rise and fall of a modern epidemic', in M. G. Marmot and P. Elliott, *Coronary Heart Disease Epidemiology: from Etiology to Public Health*, pp. 3–19, New York: Oxford University Press.
9 Kaplan, G. A. and J. E. Keil (1993), 'Socioeconomic factors and cardio-vascular disease: a review of the literature', *Circulation*, 88, pp. 1973–1998.
10 Suadicani, P., H. O. Hein and F. Gyntelberg (1997), 'Strong mediators of social inequalities in risk of ischaemic heart disease: a six-year follow-up in the Copenhagen Male Study', *International Journal of Epidemiology*, 26, pp. 516–522.
11 Morris, J. N. (1979), 'Social inequalities undiminished', *Lancet*, 1, pp. 87–90.
12 Pocock, S. J., A. G. Shaper, D. G. Cook, A. N. Phillips and M. Walker (1987), 'Social class differences in ischaemic heart disease in British men', *Lancet*, 2, pp. 197–201.
13 Marmot, M. G. (1988), 'Psychosocial factors and cardiovascular disease: epidemiological approaches', *European Heart Journal*, 9, pp. 690–697.
14 Holman, C. D. J., B. Corti, R. J. Donovan and G. Jalleh (1998), 'Association of the health-promoting workplace with trade unionism and other industrial factors', *American Journal of Health Promotion*, 12, pp. 325–334.

15 Marmot, M. G., M. J. Shipley and G. Rose (1984), 'Inequalities in death – specific explanations of a general pattern', *Lancet*, 1, pp. 1003–1006.
16 Buring, J. E., D. A. Evans, M. Fiore, B. Rosner and C. H. Hennekens (1987), 'Occupation and risk of death from coronary heart disease', *Journal of American Medical Association*, 258, pp. 791–792.
17 Marmot, M. G., G. D. Smith, S. Stansfeld, C. Patel, F. North, J. Head, I. White, E. Brunner and A. Feeney (1991), 'Health inequalities among British civil servants: the Whitehall II study', *Lancet*, 337, pp. 1387–1393.
18 Schnall, P. L., K. Belkić, P. A. Landsbergis and D. Baker (eds.) (2000), *Occupational medicine: state of the art reviews – workplace and cardiovascular disease*, Philadelphia: Hanley & Belfus.
19 Hemingway, H., H. Kuper and M. G. Marmot (2003), 'Psychosocial factors in the primary and secondary prevention of coronary heart disease: an updated systematic review of prospective cohort studies', in S. Yusuf, J. Cairns, J. Camm, E. Fallen and B. Gersch (eds), *Evidence-based cardiology*, pp. 181–218, London: British Medical Journal Publishing Group.
20 Tsutsumi, A. and N. Kawakami (2004), 'A review of empirical studies on the model of effort–reward imbalance at work: reducing occupational stress by implementing a new theory', *Social Science and Medicine*, 59, pp. 2335–2359.
21 Hallqvist, J., F. Diderichsen, T. Theorell, C. Reuterwall and A. Ahlbom (1998), 'Is the effect of job strain on myocardial infarction risk due to interaction between high psychological demands and low decision latitude? Results from Stockholm Heart Epidemiology Program (SHEEP)', *Social Science and Medicine*, 46, pp. 1405–1415.
22 Siegrist, J. and M. G. Marmot (2004), 'Health inequalities and the psychosocial environment – two scientific challenges', *Social Science and Medicine*, 58, pp. 1463–1473.
23 Bosma, H., R. Peter, J. Siegrist and M. G. Marmot (1998), 'Two alternative job stress models and the risk of coronary heart disease', *American Journal of Public Health*, 88, pp. 68–74.
24 Siegrist, J., D. Starke, T. Chandola, I. Godin, M. G. Marmot, I. Niedhammer, and R. Peter (2004), 'The measurement of effort–reward imbalance at work: European comparisons', *Social Science and Medicine*, 58, pp. 1483–1499.
25 Johnson, J. V. and E. M. Hall (1995), 'Class, work, and health' in B. C. Amick III, S. Levine, A. R. Tarlov and D. C. Walsh, *Society and Health*, pp. 247–271, New York: Oxford University Press.
26 Marmot, M. G., H. Bosma, H. Hemingway, E. Burnes and E. Stansfeld (1997), 'Contribution of job control and other risk factors to social variations in coronary heart disease incidence', *Lancet*, 350, pp. 235–239.
26 Schrijvers, C. T. M., H. D. van de Mheen, K. Stronks and J. P. Mackenbach (1998), 'Socioeconomic inequalities in health in the working population: the contribution of working conditions', *International Journal of Epidemiology*, 27, pp. 1011–1018.
28 Lynch, J., N. Krause, G. A. Kaplan, J. Tuomilehto and J. T. Salonen (1997), 'Workplace conditions, socioeconomic status, and the risk of mortality

and acute myocardial infarction: the Kuopio Ischemic Heart Disease Risk Factor Study', *American Journal of Public Health*, 87, pp. 617–622.
29. Theorell, T., A. Tsutsumi, J. Hallquist, C. Reuterwall, C. Hogstedt, P. Fredlund, N. Emlund and J. V. Johnson (1998), 'Decision latitude, job strain and myocardial infarction: a study of working men in Stockholm', *American Journal of Public Health*, 88, pp. 382–388.
30. Kivimäki, M., P. Leino-Arjas, R. Luukkonen, H. Riihimäki, J. Vahtera and J. Kirjone (2002), 'Work stress and risk of cardiovascular mortality: prospective cohort study of industrial employees', *British Medical Journal*, 325, pp. 857–860.
31. Kuper, H., A. Singh-Manoux, J. Siegrist and M. Marmot (2002), 'When reciprocity fails: effort–reward imbalance in relation to coronary heart disease and health functioning within the Whitehall II Study', *Occupational and Environmental Medicine*, 59, pp. 777–784.
32. North, F. M., S. L. Syme, A. Feeney, M. Shipley and M. Marmot (1996), 'Psychosocial work environment and sickness absence among British civil servants: the Whitehall II study', *American Journal of Public Health*, 86, pp. 322–340.
33. Ishikawa, S., T. Gotoh, N. Nago and K. Kayaba (2002), 'The Jichi Medical School (JMS) Cohort Study: design, baseline data and standardized mortality ratios', *Journal of Epidemiology*, 12, pp. 408–417.
34. Tsutsumi, A., K. Kayaba, K. Tsutsumi and M. Igarashi (2001), 'Association between job strain and prevalence of hypertension: a cross sectional analysis in a Japanese working population with a wide range of occupations: the Jichi Medical School Cohort Study', *Occupational and Environmental Medicine*, 58, pp. 367–373.
35. Tsutsumi, A., K. Tsutsumi, K. Kayaba and M. Igarashi (1998), 'Occupational status and plasma fibrinogen levels in Japanese female workers', The 5th International Congress of Behavioral Medicine, Copenhagen, Denmark.
36. International Labour Office (1990), *ISCO-88 International Standard Classification of Occupants*, Geneva: International Labour Office.
37. Tsutsumi, A. and N. Kawakami (2005), Doryoku-hōshū fukinkō sutoresu sihyō no shakai kaisō kan hikaku (Comparison of effort–reward imbalance stress indicators among social classes), The 75th Annual Meeting of the Japanese Society for Hygiene.
38. Rothman, K. J. (1986), *Modern Epidemiology*, Boston: Little, Brown.
39. Hosmer, D. W. and S. Lemeshow (1992), 'Confidence interval estimation of interaction', *Epidemiology*, 3, pp. 452–456.
40. Kawakami, N., T. Haratani, F. Kobayashi, M. Ishizaki, T. Hayashi, O. Fujita, Y. Aizawa, S. Miyazaki, H. Hiro, T. Masumoto, S. Hashimoto and S. Araki (2004), 'Occupational class and exposure to job stressors among employed men and women in Japan', *Journal of Epidemiology*, 14, pp. 204–211.
41. Tsutsumi, A., K. Kayaba, M. Nagami, A. Miki, Y. Kawano, Y. Ohya, Y. Odagiri and T. Shimomitsu (2002), 'The effort–reward imbalance model: experience in Japanese working population', *Journal of Occupational Health*, 44, pp. 398–407.
42. Andersen, I., H. Burr, T. S. Kristensen, M. Gamborg, M. Osler, E. Prescott and F. Diderichsen (2004), 'Do factors in the psychosocial work environment mediate the effect of socioeconomic position on the

risk of myocardial infarction? Study from the Copenhagen Centre for Prospective Population Studies', *Occupational and Environmental Medicine*, 61, pp. 886–892.

43 Kawakami, N., A. Tsutsumi, S. Takao, M. Ishizaki, T. Hayashi, S. Miyazaki, H. Hiro, T. Masumoto, F. Kobayashi, O. Fujita, Y. Aizawa, T. Haratani and S. Araki (2004), Shokugyō sei sutoresu wa shokugyō kaisō to utsu jōtai to no kankei wo setsumei suru ka (Does job stress explain the relation between occupational class and depressive state?), The 15th Annual Scientific Meeting of the Japan Epidemiological Association.

44 Ishizaki, M., P. Martikainen, H. Nakagawa and M. Marmot (2001), 'Socioeconomic status, workplace characteristics and plasma fibrinogen level of Japanese male employees', *Scandinavian Journal of Work, Environment and Health*, 27, pp. 287–291.

45 Kuper, H. and M. Marmot (2003), 'Job strain, job demands, decision latitude, and risk of coronary heart disease within the Whitehall II study', *Journal of Epidemiology and Community Health*, 57, pp. 147–153.

46 Vrijkotte, T. G. M., L. J. P. van Doornen and E. J. C. de Geus (1999), 'Work stress and metabolic and hemostatic risk factors', *Psychosomatic Medicine*, 61, pp. 796–805.

47 Brunner, E. J., G. D. Smith, M. Marmot, R. Canner, M. Beksinska and J. O'Brien (1996), 'Childhood social circumstances and psychosocial and behavioural factors as determinants of plasma fibrinogen', *Lancet*, 347, pp. 1008–1013.

48 Tsutsumi, A., T. Theorell, J. Hallqvist, C. Reuterwall and U. de Faire (1999). 'Association between job characteristics and plasma fibrinogen in normal working population: a cross sectional analysis on referents of the SHEEP study', *Journal of Epidemiology and Community Health*, 53, pp. 348–354.

49 Landsbergis, P. A., P. L. Schnall, T. G. Pickering, K. Warren and J. E. Schwartz (2003), 'Lower socioeconomic status among men in relation to the association between job strain and blood pressure', *Scandinavian Journal of Work, Environment and Health*, 29, pp. 206–215.

50 Pikhart, H., M. Bobak, A. Pajak, S. Malyutina, R. Kubinova, R. Topor, H. Sebakova, Y. Nikitin and M. Marmot (2004), 'Psychosocial factors at work and depression in three countries of Central and Eastern Europe', *Social Science and Medicine*, 58, pp. 1475–1482.

51 European Commission Directorate General for Employment and Social Affairs (2002), *Guidance on work-related stress: spice of life or kiss of death?*, Luxembourg: Office for Official Publications of the European Communities.

52 NORA Organization of Work Team Members (2002), *The changing organization of work and the safety and health of working people*, Cincinnati (Ohio): National Institute for Occupational Safety and Health.

53 Takao, S., N. Kawakami, T. Ohtsu and the Japan Work Stress and Health Cohort Study Group (2003), 'Occupational class and physical activity among Japanese employees', *Social Science and Medicine*, 57, pp. 2281–2289.

54 Kivimäki, M., J. Vahtera, M. Virtanen, M. Elovainio, J. Pentti and J. E. Ferrie (2003), 'Temporary employment and risk of overall and cause-specific mortality', *American Journal of Epidemiology*, 158, pp. 663–668.

55 Tsutsumi, A., K. Kayaba, T. Theorell and J. Siegrist (2001), 'Association between job stress and depression among Japanese employees threatened by job loss in a comparison between two complementary job-stress models', *Scandinavian Journal of Work, Environment and Health*, 27, pp. 146–153.

Part II
Culture, Education, Social Relationships and Health

6 Education Inequality and Health
Hiroki Sugimori

Education and health

In Western countries, socioeconomic status, which includes level of education, income and occupation, has been highlighted as one factor related to behaviour and lifestyle which leads to both social inequality and poor health[1-3]. In particular, disparity in education is a key issue, and several Western countries have taken measures to reduce this difference. In its White Paper, *Saving Lives: Our Healthier Nation*[4] (1999), the British government discussed the social determinants of health, particularly education disparities associated with health inequality, and asserted that it would take responsibility for such inequality and implement active measures to reduce it.

> 4.9 While the roots of health inequality run deep, we refuse to accept such inequality as inevitable. Moreover, we fully accept the responsibility of Government to address such deep-seated problems. That is why we are committed to a wide-ranging programme of action, right across Government, to tackle them.
>
> 4.16 Education is vital to health. People with low levels of educational achievement are more likely to have poor health as adults. So by improving education for all we will tackle one of the main causes of inequality in health...[4]

In recent years, Western countries have been focusing on disparities in literacy levels caused by education differences. Particular attention has been paid to the concept of 'health literacy'. Chapter 11 of the US government's *Healthy People 2010*[5] is entitled 'Health Communication', and focuses on communication skills related to health, as well as listing improvement in health literacy as an important goal.

Table 6.1: Definitions of health literacy

Source	Definition
Center for Health Care Strategies Inc., 2000	Health Literacy is the ability to read, understand, and act on health care information.
Special Committee on Health Literacy, American Medical Association Scientific Council, 1999	... a constellation of skills, including the ability to perform basic reading and numerical skills required to function in the health care environment.
WHO, Health Promotion Glossary, 1998	Health literacy represents the cognitive and social skills which determine the motivation and ability of individuals to gain access to, understand and use information in ways which promote and maintain good health.
U.S. National Library Service for the Blind and Physically Handicapped & Health and Human Services, 2000	The capacity to obtain, interpret and understand basic health information and services and the competence to use such information and services to enhance health. (Adopted in *Heathy People 2010*).

Below, in this chapter, I describe the concept of health literacy, which has attracted attention as a new topic in health care mainly in multilingual Western countries, but which is not yet very familiar in Japan. Then I analyse the relationship between health literacy and social structure, and that between health literacy and health outcomes.

Concept of health literacy

'Health literacy' means skills to effectively utilise information on health care, or 'reading, writing and arithmetic' skills in the field of health care. To live a healthy life in present times, it is important to digest health information accurately, and correctly understand the meanings of laboratory test values and degrees of risks. Table 6.1 is a summary of representative definitions of health literacy. The difference between health literacy and general literacy is that the former relates specifically to the field of health care only. As described below, good general literacy does not always guarantee a good understanding of concepts and terminology used in communicating health information. However, these literacies can be looked on as two sides of the same coin, and a population with low general literacy usually has low health literacy.

Improving health literacy means not only being able to understand health information more correctly, but also actively increasing opportunities to access and effectively utilise health information. The idea is that one becomes healthier through empowerment (improving the ability to control one's own life). In addition, health literacy is not limited to individual levels of literacy but more broadly, community levels. That is, improvement of health literacy not only aims to improve individual lifestyles and access to health services; it also intends to improve the level of health of the community as a whole by improving knowledge, understanding and skills. In this sense, improvement of health literacy can be regarded as part of a population-wide strategy within public health. Don Nutbeam has proposed an outcome model for health promotion (Figure 6.1). In this model, health literacy is an instrument to be made good use of in the promotion of community health and health policies, and to break down structural barriers to health[6, 7].

Furthermore, Nutbeam states that health agencies related to the WHO, whose goal is 'Health for All', should tie up with education agencies related to UNESCO, whose goal is 'Education for All'[6]. Nutbeam also encourages mass-education for the sake of improved health literacy, and argues that this is a global challenge for the twenty-first century[7]. In Japan, too, it will be essential to seek cooperation between health care practitioners and educators in the future.

Health literacy and social structure

Research into the relationship between health literacy and social structure stemmed from the results of the National Adult Literacy Survey (NALS)[8] conducted in the USA in 1992. This assessed the ability of American adults to use written texts (news articles, etc.) and reference materials (vehicle timetables, etc.). The survey showed that of 191 million American adults, approximately 40 million did not have functional literacy and another 53.5 million had a literacy level of just above the functional level. Even among high school graduates, 16% had literacy skills of level 1 (the lowest of the five literacy levels) and 36% had level 2 literacy skills. Further, 4% and 11% of all bachelor degree holders showed literacy levels of 1 and 2, respectively. These results showed that low literacy is a serious issue in the USA.

Currently, most health information in the USA is presented in literacy levels above the level of grade ten[9]. This makes it too hard

Figure 6.1: Roles of health literacy in health promotion

Health and social outcomes

Social outcomes
measures include: quality of life, functional independence, equity

Health outcomes
measures include: reduced morbidity, disability, avoidable mortality

Intermediate health outcomes (modifiable determinants of health)	Healthy lifestyle measures include: tobacco use, food choices, physical activity, alcohol and illicit drug use	Effective health services measures include: provision of preventative services, access to and appropriateness of health services	Healthy environments measures include: safe physical environments, supportive economic and social conditions, good food supply, restricted access to tobacco, alcohol
Health promotion outcomes (intervention impact measures)	Health literacy measures include: health-related knowledge, attitudes, motivation, bewhavioural intentions, personal skills, self-efficacy	Social action and influence measures include: community participation, community empowerment, social norms, public opinion	Healthy public policy and organizational practice measures include: policy statements, legislation, regulation, resource allocation, organizational practices
Health promotion actions	Education examples include: patient education, school education, broadcast media and print media education	Social mobilization examples include: community development, group facilitation, targeted mass communication	Advocacy examples include: lobbying, political organization, overcoming bureaucratic inertia

Source: Nutbeam (2000)[6]. Reproduced with permission from Oxford University Press.

for many American adults to fully understand health information provided by physicians, pharmacists, public health nurses, other health care professionals and pharmaceutical companies (e.g. in package inserts, etc.). In addition, it has been reported that low literacy is associated with poor health status in American adults. Under these circumstances, the concept of health literacy has been mentioned in recent years as functional literacy, specifically for the field of health care. Table 6.2 is a summary of previous

US studies on the relationship between health literacy and social structure, arranged in chronological order.

The elderly

There have been a number of reports showing low health literacy among the elderly[10–12]. One study has assessed health literacy of Medicare (public health insurance for the elderly) recipients using the English and Spanish TOFHLA (Test of Functional Health Literacy in Adults). The results showed a significantly strong association between old age and low health literacy. This association remained significant after adjustment for the numbers of years of education and cognitive level[11]. An association with low health literacy has also been reported among emergency patients at urban public hospitals[12], hypertensive patients, diabetic patients[13], emergency outpatients and asthmatic outpatients[14], affluent retirees[15] and type II diabetic patients[16]. The elderly account for a large proportion of medical costs. From the perspective of ensuring more appropriate medical expenditure, improvement of health literacy among the elderly is an important issue and an area for intervention in Japan as well.

Minority groups, immigrants and ethnic groups

The NALS showed low literacy in many Hispanic and African residents in the USA. More recent studies have reported low literacy and low health literacy in minority groups, including non-Caucasian[16, 17], Hispanic[12, 14, 19] and African residents[20, 21].

Hispanic residents are currently the most rapidly increasing ethnic group in the USA. The US population survey data for 2000 (US & World 2001) estimates that Hispanic residents increased by 58% during the 1990s to 35.3 million, accounting for 12.5% of the entire US population. Currently, the Hispanic population is said to be the largest ethnic group of the US minority groups, outnumbering the African-American population. Unlike traditional Hispanic residents, they have low education attainment levels (education status). While traditional Hispanic residents used to be distributed mainly in Texas, California and Florida, new Hispanic residents have been increasing particularly in North Carolina, Georgia, Arkansas, Tennessee, South Carolina, Alabama and Kentucky, where the numbers of Spanish-speaking public servants are limited, resulting in insufficient public support for these residents.

Table 6.2: Previous studies on health literacy and social structure

Reference	Year	Study population	Health literacy assessment tool	Social structural factors associated with low health literacy
Weiss, et al.[18]	1994	N = 402. Medicaid enrollees (average age, 49 years).	IDL	Spanish-speaking population.
Williams, et al.[12]	1995	N = 2659. Patients who arrived for emergency treatment. 1892 English-speaking and 767 Spanish-speaking subjects (Literacy in Health Care study).	TOFHLA	Spanish-speaking population above 60 years of age.
Bennett, et al.[19]	1998	N = 212. African Americans (average age, 70.8 years).	REALM	Being African-American, region (Louisiana).
Williams, et al.[13, 14]	1998	N = 483. Emergency department patients (273; average age, 37 years), asthma outpatients (210; average age, 47 years).	REALM	Being elderly.
Williams, et al.[14]	1998	N = 516. Hypertensive patients (402), diabetic patients (114).	TOFHLA	Being elderly, Spanish-speaking population.
Gazmararian, et al.[10]	1999	N = 406. Women registered with Medicaid. Age distribution: 19-24 years (144), 25-29 years (86), 30 years (175).	TOFHLA (simplified version)	Low education level and low health literacy level had no clear relationship with age, race, marital status, employment status or poverty.
Gazmararian, Parker & Baker[31]	1999	N = 3260. New Medicare enrollees (Prudential Medicare Managed Care Study).	S-TOFHLA	Being African-American, being elderly, a short school education, being blue-collar and old age were strongly associated with low health literacy. The association remained significant after adjustment for education and cognition level.

Reference	Year	Study population	Health literacy assessment tool	Social structural factors associated with low health literacy
Kalichman, et al.[22]	2000	N = 228. HIV+ adults (average age, 39.7 years)	TOFHLA	Short school education, ethnic minority, health literacy level had no association with age, income level, gender or sexual orientation (homosexual).
Arnold, et al.[20]	2001	N = 600. Pregnant women. Caucasian (303), African-American (296).	REALM	Being African-American.
Benson & Forman[15]	2002	N = 93. Male (22), female (71). Average age, 83 years.	TOFHLA	Old age, short education.
Lindau, et al.[17]	2002	N = 529. English-speaking patients over 18 years of age. Average age, 27 years.	REALM	Non-Caucasian subjects, those who carry no insurance or carry public insurance.
Schillinger, et al.[16]	2002	N = 408. English- and Spanish-speaking type II diabetic patients over 30 years of age (San Francisco General Diabetic Patients with Low Health Literacy Study).	S-TOFHLA	Being elderly, female, non-Caucasian, Spanish-speaking population, low education level, Medicare patients, patients with long-term diabetes.
Beers, et al.[21]	2003	N = 1805. African-American, 58%; male, 66% (Health Literacy Satisfaction Study).	REALM	Being African-American, being elderly, a low education level. After adjustment for education level, old age had no association while race remained potentially associated with low health literacy.

Education attainment levels, years of education and education status

People with limited education usually have limited general literacy. The NALS results showed that more than 80% of those who did not finish high school had literacy skills of NALS level 1 or 2. While further studies are warranted for health literacy levels in populations with limited education, it has been believed that poor health literacy often exists where there is poor general literacy, as in the present situation[15, 16, 21, 22].

Low income

Low income correlates with low literacy, old age, being a member of a racial/ethnic minority, a low education attainment level, being an immigrant and/or other social structure factors. It has not been conclusively determined whether low literacy results in low income or results from a lack of opportunities for education due to social structure circumstances. However, a number of reports have suggested an association between poor general literacy and poor health literacy among low-income classes. In a study of 402 Hispanic Medicaid recipients (public health insurance for low-income earners and a valid surrogate variable for low-income classes in the USA), the average literacy level was about the level of grade five, and one-fifth of the patients had a literacy level of about grade two[18]. In another study which analysed low-income emergency outpatients at two urban public hospitals, a significant association was found between poor health literacy and being a Hispanic resident. 50% of the patients were unable to understand the dosage instructions, and 60% were unable to understand a standard informed consent form[12].

Health literacy and health outcomes

A large number of studies have been reported from the USA on the association between health literacy and health outcomes (health status and use of health care service). Table 6.3 is a summary of reports on health literacy and health outcomes, arranged in chronological order.

Figure 6.2 shows hypothetical pathways between health literacy and health outcomes based on reports from the USA.[23] This figure has four intervening variables (interim outcomes): knowledge about disease and self-care; health risk avoidance behaviour (lifestyles); preventive care and regular access to physicians; and drug compliance. The final outcomes are health status, emergency care and in-patient care.

Within these pathways, people with low health literacy would have poor knowledge of disease and self-care. This tends to result in poor lifestyles and a failure to engage in health risk avoidance behaviour. In addition, these people would be unable to correctly understand physicians' instructions and information contained in appointment sheets or letters of referral. This would result in poorer participation in vaccinations and other preventive programs, and fewer people seeing physicians regularly. Furthermore, they would have poor drug compliance (an inability to take prescribed drugs in accordance with the instructions). As a result, they would be unable to benefit from preventive or health care services in a timely, appropriate manner. It follows that these people would tend to have poor health status and their diseases become serious, resulting in more need for emergency or in-patient medical care. Such is the idea hypothesised in Figure 6.2.

In this figure, the links between health literacy and intervening variables are simplified. To be more accurate, it is necessary to make appropriate adjustments for confounding factors, including social structure factors (e.g. socioeconomic status, education attainment level, age, gender, race, US health insurance coverage, disease severity, income disparity and ethnic composition). Also omitted from the figure are interactions among intervening variables and feedback on the final outcomes. For instance, a person who has a severe disease and frequently uses in-patient care may learn to make good use of medical information through his/her experience and obtain a high level of health literacy[23].

Knowledge of disease, self-care and health risk avoidance

People with low health literacy tend to have poor knowledge of diseases and thus have poor ability to take care of themselves properly. They tend to have poor knowledge of chronic diseases[24] and tend to use preventive services infrequently[13, 25–27]. People with low health literacy tend to have poor knowledge of the adverse effects of smoking[20], hypertension and diabetes[13], breast cancer risk[28], the severity of children's diseases[29], asthma knowledge scores[14], cervical cancer screening[30], contraception[31] and HIV therapies[32].

There are only a small number of studies that have conducted detailed analyses of the association between health literacy and health risk avoidance behaviour. Individuals with low health literacy have

Table 6.3: Previous studies on health literacy and health outcomes

Reference	Year	Study population	Health literacy assessment tool	Analytical methods for health outcomes	Health outcomes associated with health literacy
Williams, et al.[12]	1995	N = 2659. Poor people, minority patients, English-speaking patients (1982), Spanish-speaking patients (767).	TOFHLA		People with low health literacy tended not to comply with physicians' instructions and had difficulty understanding appointment sheets or letters of referral.
Baker, et al.[35]	1997	N = 2659. Atlanta, Los Angeles (979), English-speaking population (913), Spanish-speaking population (767) (Literacy in Health Care Study).	TOFHLA	Interviews	Low as compared to high health literacy was significantly associated with complaints of poor health. This association remained after adjustment for age, gender, race and socioeconomic indicators.
Baker, et al.[41]	1998	N = 979 (Literacy in Health Care Study).	S-TOFHLA	Structural interviews, Grady Memorial Hospital information system.	The average frequency of admission to emergency departments was higher in patients with low health literacy than those with high health literacy by a factor of more than one. This association remained after adjustment for age, gender, race, self-reported health status and other socioeconomic status and health insurance coverage.
Bennett, et al.[19]	1998	N = 212. Low-income earners: African-American (109), Caucasian (103) (average age, 70.8 years)	REALM	Medical record review, pathological reports.	Low as compared to high health literacy was significantly associated with first hospital visit only after cancer had reached an advanced stage (stage D).
Moon, et al.[29]	1998	N = 543. Parents bringing children to clinics (average age, 32 years)	REALM	Interviews	Health literacy was significantly associated with parental understanding of disease severity in their children.
Williams, et al.[14]	1998	N = 483. Emergency department (273; average age, 37 years), asthma clinic (210; average age, 47 years)	REALM	Interviews, observation of use of asthma medication metered dose inhalers (MDIs).	Patients with low literacy had low asthma knowledge scores. Patients with low ability to read and comprehend had low skill to use MDIs.
Williams, et al.[13]	1998	N = 518. patients (402), diabetic patients (114).	TOFHLA (in either English or Spanish)	Interviews	Patients with low or borderline health literacy had poor knowledge about hypertension or diabetes (hypoglycemic symptoms).

Reference	Year	Study population	Health literacy assessment tool	Analytical methods for health outcomes	Health outcomes associated with health literacy
Gazmararian, Parker & Baker[31]	1999	N = 406. Women registered with health plan. Age distribution: 19-24 years (144), 25-29 years (86), 30 years (175).	S-TOFHLA	Interviews	Women with low health literacy: use for contraceptive purposes intrauterine device (IUD), douche, rhythm method (Ogino method) and contraceptive pills (levonorgestrel) more often than other methods; wish to know 4.4 times as many contraceptive methods; and tend to have inaccurate knowledge about contraception during years when they are prone to becoming pregnant. These associations remained significant after adjustment for age, race and marital status.
Kalichman, Ramachandran & Catz[27]	1999	N = 182. HIV+ adults (average age, 39.1 years).	Adapted reading comprehension section of TOFHLA		HIV+ adults with low health literacy are more prone to making mistakes in the amounts of AIDS drugs than those with high health literacy.
Gazmararian et al.[36]	2000	N = 3260. New Medicare enrollees, English-speaking subjects (2956), Spanish-speaking subjects (304).	S-TOFHLA	Geriatric Depression Scale (GDS), interviews.	People with low health literacy more often had depression. This association did not remain significant after adjustment for health status.
Kalichman & Rompa[34]	2000	N = 339. HIV+ adults (average age, 40 years).	Part of TOFHLA (reading comprehension test)		HIV carriers with low health literacy: had fewer CD4 cells and higher amounts of virus; more often failed to take antiretroviral agents; were more often hospitalised; and more often had poor health status.
Kalichman, et al.[22]	2000	N = 228. HIV+ adults (average age, 40 years).	TOFHLA	Questionnaires or interviews	Those with low health literacy: less often had undetectable levels of virus; less often understood the meaning of CD4 cell counts; were more often asked questions by their physicians about their treatment; and more often received explanations from their physicians.
Arnold, et al.[20]	2001	N = 600. Pregnant women: Caucasian (303), African-American (296).	REALM	Urinary nicotine level, self-reported smoking habit survey.	Those with low health literacy had poorer knowledge about adverse effects of smoking and had less concern over effects of smoking on children.
Fortenberry, et al.[38]	2001	N = 1035. Average age, 26 years.	REALM	Structural interviews.	Those with low health literacy more often had positive gonorrhoea test results.

Table 6.3: continued

Reference	Year	Study population	Health literacy assessment tool	Analytical methods for health outcomes	Health outcomes associated with health literacy
Kaufman, et al.[59]	2001	N = 61. First-time mothers over 18 years old who spoke English as their mother tongue and had children between 2 and 12 months of age.	REALM		Participants with high health literacy more often started breastfeeding during the first 2 months and continued breastfeeding thereafter.
Baker, et al.[39]	2002	N = 3260. Medicare enrollees: English-speaking subjects (2956), Spanish-speaking subjects (304) (Prudential Medicare Managed Care Study).	S-TOFHLA	Structural interviews, Mini Mental State Examination (MMSE), GDS, Short Form 12 (SF-12), self-reported psychosomatic assessment scores, application for managed care.	Enrollees with low health literacy had poorer health status and were significantly more often hospitalised than those with high health literacy. This association remained after adjustment for demographic variables, income, school education, cognitive functions and social support.
Baker, et al.[37]	2002	N = 2787. Medicare enrollees: Caucasian (2343), African-American (354) (average age, 73 years) (Prudential Medicare Managed Care Study).	S-TOFHLA	MMSE, self-reports.	A correlation was found between health literacy and total MMSE score.
Gordon, et al.[57]	2002	N = 123. Patients with chronic rheumatoid arthritis (average age, 37 years; range, 19 to 77 years)	REALM	Interviews, medical history review, Health Anxiety Questionnaire (HAQ) and Hospital Anxiety and Depression Scale (HADS) scores, Carstairs index of social deprivation.	Patients with low health literacy consulted at hospitals 3 times more often than control subjects during the past 12 months.
Lindau, et al.[17]	2002	N = 529. English-speaking patients over 18 years of age (average age, 27 years): African-American (58%), Hispanic (18%).	REALM	Interviews, medical record review, physician survey.	Health literacy was significantly associated with knowledge about cervical cancer screening.

Education Inequality and Health

Reference	Year	Study population	Health literacy assessment tool	Analytical methods for health outcomes	Health outcomes associated with health literacy
Schillinger, et al.[16]	2002	N = 408. English- and Spanish-speaking type II diabetic patients over 30 years of age (San Francisco General Diabetic Patients with Low Health Literacy Study).	S-TOFHLA	Diabetic care profile social support scale, short form of CES-D, interviews, hospital databases.	Health literacy was associated with HbA1c level after adjustment for social factors, depression, social support, treatment regimen and years of diabetes. Patients with low health literacy had poor blood-sugar control and a high incidence of diabetic retinopathy.
Scott, et al.[25]	2002	N = 2722. New Medicare enrollees between 65 and 80 years of age (average age, 71 years) (Prudential Medicare Managed Care Study).	S-TOFHLA	Interviews	People with low health literacy less often used preventive health services (influenza and pneumococcal vaccination, mammography and Pap smear).
Guerra & Shea[40]	2003	N = 1301. Patients over 18 years of age who had Medicaid or Medicare coverage (average age, 42.2 years) (Health Literacy and Patient Satisfaction Study).	TOFHLA	Charlson Comorbidity Index, SF-12.	Patients with low health literacy more frequently had complications after adjustment for counfounding factors.
Schillinger, et al.[58]	2003	N = 74. English-speaking, low-health literacy diabetic patients (average age, 64 years; Caucasian, 85%) (San Francisco General Diabetic Patients with Low Health Literacy Study).	S-TOFHLA	Tape recordings of dialogues between patients and physicians.	High health literacy and physicians' interactive communication policy were two factors associated with good blood-sugar control.
Weiss & Palmer[62]	2004	Arizona's managed-Medicaid plan, the Arizona Health Care Cost Containment System (AHCCCS).	IDR		Average annual medical expense was $10,688 and $2891 for Medicaid recipients with low health literacy and those with high health literacy, respectively.

Figure 6.2: Schematic diagram of a model of associations between health literacy and health outcomes

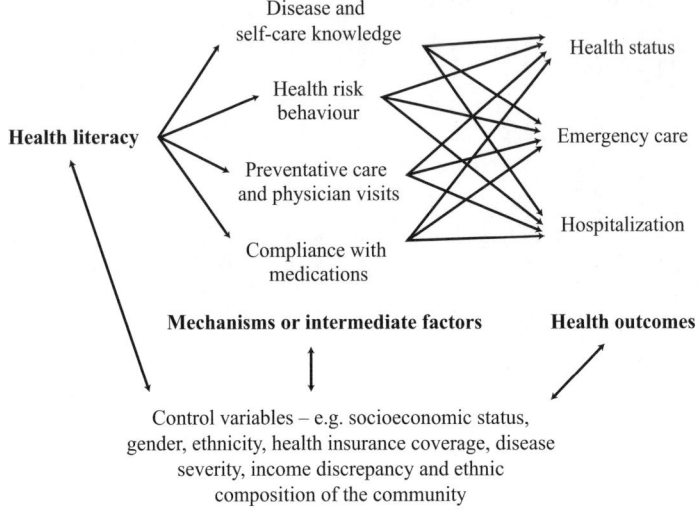

Source: partially modified by the author from Lee, Arozullah & Cho (2004)[23].

a strong tendency toward lifestyles that include smoking, alcohol consumption, abuse of illegal drugs, little physical activity and so on, and tend not to adopt health risk avoidance behaviour. This is thought to have been because low health literacy is associated with fewer opportunities to improve an individual's ability to understand health and medical information. In addition, individuals with low health literacy tend to be sceptical about medical instructions. This seems to make it hard for them to make lifestyle changes, such as adopting health risk avoidance behaviour.

Preventive care and access to physicians

People with low health literacy tend to have a poor understanding of, and less access to, information on the importance of the early detection and early treatment of disease. They have poorer voluntary participation in decision-making on health care and tend to use preventive care infrequently. They tend to have poor understanding of physicians' explanations or of information provided in appointment sheets or letters of referral[12], and tend to receive periodic checkups less often. Low health literacy is associated with less frequent use of preventive health services (e.g. for influenza and pneumococcal vaccination, mammography and Pap smear checks)[25] and less frequent outpatient visits[33].

Drug compliance

It has been reported that low health literacy is associated with low drug compliance. Asthma patients with low health literacy tend to have poor skills for using asthma medication, such as metered dose inhalers (MDIs)[14]. In outpatient clinics specialising in HIV care and AIDS service agencies, HIV-positive patients with low health literacy have been reported to make mistakes more often in the amounts of medication[27]. In addition, a larger proportion of them fail to take antiretroviral drugs[34].

Health status

People with low health literacy more often report poor health than those with high health literacy[35]. Those with low health literacy report depression more often[36]. A correlation has been found between health literacy and total MMSE scores[37]. Furthermore, HIV carriers with low health literacy tend to have fewer CD4 cells and higher amounts of HIV virus[34]. People with low health literacy more often have positive gonorrhoea test results[39]. Medicare recipients with low health literacy often have poorer health status[39]. In the context of diabetes, health literacy is associated with HbA1c levels. Diabetic patients with low health literacy tend to have poorer blood-sugar control and a higher incidence of diabetic retinopathy[16] and of complications[40].

Emergency and in-patient care

Patients with low health literacy are admitted to an emergency department more often than those with high health literacy by a factor of more than one[41]. Also, among Medicare recipients, patients with low health literacy are more frequently hospitalised than those with high health literacy [39], and there is a similar trend for HIV carriers[34].

Medical expenses

Medicaid is public health insurance for the elderly in the USA, and in 1992, the annual average medical expenses for Medicaid recipients with low health literacy and those with high health literacy were $10,688 and $2,891, respectively[42]. In particular, hospital expenses differed greatly between recipients with low health literacy (an annual amount of $7,038) and those with high literacy ($824). Similar results have been obtained among Medicare recipients. Compared to Medicare recipients with sufficient literacy, those with low health literacy incurred higher expenses for emergency care, prescription drugs and hospital care by $86, $137 and $1,107, respectively, in each case on an annual basis[43].

Assessment of health literacy

Representative tools for health literacy assessment are shown in Table 6.4[44]. Of the tools shown, the word comprehension test, TOFHLA[45], and the word recognition test, REALM[46], are representative.

A word comprehension test assesses the ability to read and comprehend written text. TOFHLA (Test of Functional Health Literacy in Adults) is a well-known cloze test. A cloze test is a form of test that uses text with some of its words replaced with blanks in a systematic manner and requests subjects to fill in the blanks. It is a so-called fill-in-the-blanks test. TOFHLA is based on the hypothesis that subjects with higher literacy better understand the text and are thus better able to fill in the blanks in the text. It was developed to help research into health literacy in American health care settings. It comprises two sections: a reading comprehension test and a numerical ability test. The reading comprehension test section has fifty items and includes instructions for the upper digestive tract, the 'rights and responsibilities' section of a Medicaid application form, and an informed consent form. The numerical ability test section comprises seventeen items which assess the ability to comprehend seventeen numerical concepts. These numbers include those used on drug container labels, on consultation appointment sheets, and for blood-sugar levels. TOFHLA requires higher literacy than the word comprehension tests described below. It is a time-consuming assessment and is not suited for health literacy assessment in clinics or community settings.

A word recognition test is a method of assessment that requires subjects to read words aloud. It hypothesises that subjects who have problems with the basic skill of word pronunciation have low literacy. A word recognition test uses different word lists of varying

Table 6.4: List of representative tools for health literacy assessment

	Word comprehension test			Word recognition test			
	TOFHLA	S-TOFHLA	IDL	WRAT-R3	SORT-R	REALM	LAD
Type	Cloze test on the ability to comprehend health care materials	Cloze test on the ability to comprehend health care materials. Short version of TOFHLA	Reading comprehension test.	Word recognition test.	Word recognition test.	Health vocabulary recognition test.	Diabetes vocabulary recognition test
Time	18 to 22 min.	7 min.	22 min.	3 to 5 min.	5 to 10 min.	2 to 3 min.	3 to 5 min.
Scoring	Health literacy: inadequate, marginal, functional.	Health literacy: inadequate, marginal, functional.	Health literacy: inadequate, marginal, functional.	Several scores can be calculated. Scores can be converted into grade levels and standardised to specific age groups.	0 to 200 points. Raw scores can be converted into 10 different grade groups (pre-1 through combined group of grades 9 to 12)	0 to 66 points. Raw scores can be converted into 4 grade categories (grades 3 and under; grades 4 to 6; grades 7 to 8; grades 9 and over)	0 to 60 points. Raw scores can be converted into 3 grade categories
Subjects	Adults only.		All ages.	5 to 74 years.	4 years and over.	Adults only.	Adults only.
Main advantages	Spanish version can be used in Spanish-speaking populations. Functional health literacy can be assessed.		Spanish version can be used in Spanish-speaking populations.	Can be used with minors.†	Can be used in schools and workplaces.	Simple and less demanding on subjects. Large font version is available.	Simple. Can be used for diabetic education.
Main limitations	Long version is time-consuming, not simple and burdensome on subjects.		Long version is time-consuming, not simple and burdensome on subjects.	Words used are somewhat too hard for patients.	Small font size. Difficult to assess levels above grade 9.	Difficult to assess levels above grade 9. Assessment can be made only for grade groups and not for specific grades.	Insufficient evidence to support clinical application.
Other	Very short version is also available. Correlation: WRAT-3, 0.74; REALM, 0.84.		Correlation: WRAT-3, 0.74; REALM, 0.84.	Correlation: REALM, 0.88; TOFHLA, 0.74; IDL, 0.74.	Correlation: SORT-R, 0.96.	Correlation: WRAT-3, 0.88; SORT-R, 0.96; TOFHLA, 0.84; IDL, 0.84.	Correlation: WRAT-3, 0.81; REALM, 0.90.

degrees of difficulty, which contain simple to complicated words. Assessment is continued until the subject can no longer pronounce some of the words on the list. As such, a word recognition test requires only a short time in making assessments and the scoring is easy. Representative word recognition tests include WRAT-3 (Wide Range Achievement Test-3) and REALM (Rapid Estimate of Adult Literacy in Medicine). The REALM test was developed to assess literacy in health care and contains more words than the WRAT that are commonly used to describe physical and medical conditions. In the REALM test, words are presented in ascending order of difficulty so that subjects will not lose confidence. It is particularly useful in screening for individuals with low literacy.

Health literacy issues in Japan

In recent years, research into education disparities has attracted attention in Japan[47–49]. At the same time, studies into the association between education disparities and health outcomes have been increasing in number. For example, a study which analysed social inequality among the elderly reported a significant association between education history (which was used as a surrogate variable for the standard level of knowledge about health and was analysed as a binary variable of whether the subject had 'up to compulsory education' or 'higher education') and both subjective and objective health measures as indicated by the Tokyo Metropolitan Institute of Gerontology index of competence[50]. Also, the Aichi Gerontological Evaluation Study reported that the proportion of subjects who engaged in unhealthy behaviour (smoking, habitual alcohol consumption, lack of exercise and failure to undergo medical checkups) or who had a history of falls was significantly higher among the group of subjects with a short (poor) education than the group of subjects with a long education[51]. It has also been reported that depression[52] and social withdrawal[53] were more frequently seen in people with a shorter education.

In the aforementioned Aichi study of the elderly, education history was shown to have a significant association with 'social contact' or personal networks[54]. This shows that education history is related to social capital in the context of 'personal relationships', such as social participation or information access. It will be necessary to introduce the element of health literacy to the analysis of the interrelation between education and health outcomes in Japan.

Japan has maintained high levels of education, as seen in the fact that Japanese high school students rank second only in the world to Korean students in scientific knowledge[55]. In addition, being a non-multiethnic country unlike the USA, Japan has a high literacy rate and seems to have fewer health literacy problems than the USA. Still, in reality, disparities in literacy skills do seem to exist among Japanese people. It is thus necessary for Japanese researchers to analyse the possibility that disparities in health literacy may result in differences in the effects of health care. In this regard, previous American studies and approaches to health literacy are highly informative.

As mentioned above, old age is associated with low health literacy. This is an important consideration in Japan, which has a society aging even more rapidly than the USA. Coupled with the high health care needs of the elderly, low health literacy among the elderly makes them the population requiring the most attention. Information that is attractive and easy-to-understand for younger people is not always easy-to-understand for older people. There have not been sufficient studies on the methods and contents of preventive guidance and health care instructions given to the elderly. In brochures distributed to provide health information, for instance, there has hardly been any discussion of font sizes, colours, figures and tables in terms of what is most appropriate for the elderly. In this regard, the Canadian Ministry of Health's *Communicating with Seniors: Advice, Techniques and Tips*[56], issued in the International Year of Older Persons, 1999, is useful.

The development of information technology (IT) in recent years has revolutionised individuals' capacities to collect and manage information. Computers are contemporary 'abacuses' and computer skills are related to health literacy. Collection of health information through the Internet is of particular significance. While there are problems in the management of reliability and accuracy of information distributed through the Internet, it is easily conceivable that whether or not individuals have access to the Internet would result in disparities among them in their knowledge of disease, self-care and lifestyle improvements. 'Health Communication', Chapter 11 of the US government's *Healthy People 2010*, lists as one of its objectives to 'Increase the proportion of households with access to the Internet at home'. Older people who are not familiar with IT are likely to be affected more severely in their health literacy. It is necessary to pay attention to the elderly in terms of both advanced age and lack of IT skills. At the present time, when IT skills have not been widely spread among the elderly, there is concern that a 'digital divide' may directly result in a 'health divide'.

Most of the health literacy assessment tools developed in the USA are intended to assess literacy itself. In Japan, where the illiteracy rate is low, it is difficult to use these American assessment tools as they are. For example, the diversity of languages spoken in the USA is one difference that needs considering. The US Spanish-speaking Hispanic population is known to have a discrepancy between word recognition ability and literacy. Many of the word recognition tests, including REALM, examine word pronunciation based on the assumption that pronunciation ability levels are positively associated with literacy levels. However, the Spanish language is characterised by phoneme-grapheme (or sound-to-mark) correspondence, which means that phonemes correspond to letters. (In this type of language, one can pronounce words without knowing their meanings. This makes REALM and other word recognition tests, which mainly assess pronunciation, unusable in the Japanese syllabaries, including hiragana.) This makes Spanish word pronunciation relatively easy and makes it difficult to assess Spanish literacy solely by word recognition tests. This is not unrelated to the fact that no Spanish versions have been developed for REALM and other word recognition tests, while TOFHLA does have Spanish versions. The Japanese hiragana and katakana syllabaries are also characterised by phoneme-grapheme correspondence. This requires special consideration in developing tools for health literacy assessment in Japan.

Japan has high literacy, and most of its people seem to have high health literacy. In addition to the rapid aging and advanced IT development, however, Japan is likely to face many other health literacy issues in the near future. These issues will include an increase of foreign immigrants and reforms of the health care system. Japan is another country where further studies are awaited on health literacy and related issues.

Acknowledgment

The author would like to thank Dr. Shoou-Yih D. Lee of the North Carolina University, who gave much advice on the manuscript.

Literature

1 Lantz, P. M., J. S. House, J. M. Lepkowski, D. R. Williams, R. P. Mero and J. Chen (1998), 'Socioeconomic factors, health behaviors, and mortality:

results from a nationally representative prospective study of US adults', *Journal of the American Medical Association*, 279 (21), pp. 1703–1708.
2. Varo, J. J., M. A. Martinez-Gonzalez, J. De Irala-Estevez, J. Kearney, M. Gebney and J. A. Martinez (2003), 'Distribution and determinants of sedentary lifestyles in the European Union', *International Journal of Epidemiology*, 32 (1), pp. 138–146.
3. Marmot, M. G. and R. G. Wilkinson (eds.) (1999), *Social Determinants of Health*, 1st edition, Oxford: Oxford University Press.
4. Department of Health, UK (1999), *Saving Lives: Our Healthier Nation*, London: HMSO, http://www.archive.official-documents.co.uk/document/cm43/4386/4386-04.htm.
5. Department of Health and Human Services (2000), *Healthy People 2010*, Washington D.C.: DHHS, http://www.health.gov/healthypeople/document/html/volume1/11healthcom.htm
6. Nutbeam, D. (2000), 'Health literacy as a public health goal: a challenge for contemporary health education and communication strategies into the 21st century', *Health Promotion International*, 15 (3), pp. 259–267.
7. Nutbeam, D. and I. Kickbusch (2000), 'Advancing health literacy: a global challenge for the 21st century', *Health Promotion International*, 15 (3), pp. 183–184.
8. Kirsch, I. S., A. Jungeblat, L. Jenkins and A. Kolstad (1993), *Adult literacy in America: a first look at the results of the National Adult Literacy Survey*, Washington D.C.: National Center for Educational Statistics, U.S. Department of Education.
9. Davis, T. C., M. A. Crouch, G. Wills, S. Miller and D. M. Abdehou (1990), 'The gap between patient reading comprehension and the readability of patient education materials', *Journal of Family Practice*, 31 (5), pp. 533–538.
10. Gazmararian, J. A., D. W. Baker, M. V. Williams, R. M. Parker, T. L. Scott, D. C. Green, S. N. Fehrenbach, J. Ren and J. P. Koplan (1999), 'Health literacy among Medicare enrollees in a managed care organization', *Journal of the American Medical Association*, 281 (6), pp. 545–551.
11. Baker, D. W., J. A. Gazmararian, J. Sudano and M. Patterson (2000), 'The association between age and health literacy among elderly persons', *Journal of Gerontology Series B: Psychological Sciences and Social Sciences*, 55 (6), S368–374.
12. Williams, M. V., R. M. Parker, D. W. Baker, N. S. Parikh, K. Pitkin, W. C. Coates and J. R. Nurss (1995), 'Inadequate functional health literacy among patients at two public hospitals', *Journal of the American Medical Association*, 274 (21), pp. 1677–1682.
13. Williams, M. V., D. W. Baker, R. M. Parker and J. R. Nurss (1998), 'Relationship of functional health literacy to patients' knowledge of their chronic disease: a study of patients with hypertension and diabetes', *Archives of Internal Medicine*, 158 (2), pp. 166–172.
14. Williams, M. V., D. W. Baker, E. G. Honig, T. M. Lee and A. Nowlan (1998), 'Inadequate literacy is a barrier to asthma knowledge and self-care', *Chest*, 114 (4), pp. 1008–1015.
15. Benson, J. G. and W. B. Forman (2002), 'Comprehension of written health care information in an affluent geriatric retirement community: use of the Test of Functional Health Literacy', *Gerontology*, 48, pp. 93–97.

16 Schillinger, D., K. Grumbach, J. Piette, F. Wang, D. Osmond, C. Daher, J. Palacios, G. Diaz Sullivan and A. B. Bindman (2002), 'Association of health literacy with diabetes outcomes', *Journal of the American Medical Association*, 288 (4), pp. 475–482.

17 Lindau, S. T., C. Tomori, T. Lyons, L. Langseth, C. L. Bennett and P. Garcia (2002), 'The association of health literacy with cervical cancer prevention knowledge and health behaviors in a multiethnic cohort of women', *American Journal of Obstetrics and Gynecology*, 186 (5), pp. 938–943.

18 Weiss, B. D., J. S. Blanchard, D. L. McGee, G. Hart, B. Warren, M. Burgoon and K. J. Smith (1994), 'Illiteracy among Medicaid recipients and its relationship to health care costs', *Journal of Health Care for the Poor and Underserved*, 5 (2), pp. 99–111.

19 Bennett, C. L., M. R. Ferreira, T. C. Davis, J. Kaplan, M. Weinberger, T. Kuzel, M. A. Seday and O. Sartor (1998), 'Relation between literacy, race, and stage of presentation among low-income patients with prostate cancer', *Journal of Clinical Oncology*, 16 (9), pp. 3101–3104.

20 Arnold, C. L., T. C. Davis, H. J. Berkel, R. H. Jackson, I. Nandy and S. London (2001), 'Smoking status, reading level, and knowledge of tobacco effects among low-income pregnant women', *Preventive Medicine*, 32 (4), pp. 313–320.

21 Beers, B. B., V. J. McDonald, D. A. Quistberg, K. L. Ravenell, D. A. Asch and J. A. Ahea (2003), 'Disparities in health literacy between African and non-African American primary care patients', *Journal of General Internal Medicine*, 18 (Supplement 1), p. 169.

22 Kalichman, S. C., E. Benotsch, T. Suarez, S. Catz, J. Miller and D. Rompa (2000), 'Health literacy and health-related knowledge among persons living with HIV/AIDS', *American Journal of Preventive Medicine*, 18 (4), pp. 325–331.

23 Lee, S-Y. D., A. Arozullah and Y. I. Cho (2004), 'Health literacy, social support, and health: a research agenda', *Social Science and Medicine*, 58 (7), pp. 1309–1321.

24 Gazmararian, J. A., M. V. Williams, J. Peel and D. W. Baker (2003), 'Health literacy and knowledge of chronic disease', *Patient Education and Counseling*, 51 (3), pp. 267–275.

25 Scott, T. L., J. A. Gazmararian, M. V. Williams and D. W. Baker (2002), 'Health literacy and preventive health care use among Medicare enrollees in a managed care organization', *Medical Care*, 40 (5), pp. 395–404.

26 Davis, T. C., C. L. Arnold, H. J. Berkel, I. Nandy and R. H. Jackson (1996), 'Knowledge and attitude on screening mammography among low-literate, low-income women', *Cancer*, 78 (9), pp. 1912–1920.

26 Kalichman, S. C., B. Ramachandran and S. Catz (1999), 'Adherence to combination antiretroviral therapies in HIV patients of low health literacy', *Journal of General Internal Medicine*, 14 (5), pp. 267–273.

28 Jones, A. R., C. J. Thompson, R. A. Oster, A. Samadi, M. K. Davis, R. M. Mayberry and L. S. Caplan (2003), 'Breast cancer knowledge, beliefs, and screening behaviors among low-income, elderly black women', *Journal of the National Medical Association*, 95 (9), pp. 791–797, 802–805.

29 Moon, R. Y., T. L. Cheng, K. M. Patel, K. Baumhaft and P. C. Scheidt (1998), 'Parental literacy level and understanding of medical information', *Pediatrics*, 102 (2), e25.

30 Sharp, L. K., J. M. Zurawski, P. Y. Roland, C. O'Toole and J. Hines (2002), 'Health literacy, cervical cancer risk factors, and distress in low-income African-American women seeking colposcopy', *Ethnicity and Disease*, 12 (4), pp. 541–546.
31 Gazmararian, J. A., R. M. Parker and D. W. Baker (1999), 'Reading skills and family planning knowledge and practices in a low-income managed-care population', *Obstetrics and Gynecology*, 93 (2), pp. 239–244.
32 Van Servellen, G., J. S. Brown, E. Lombardi, G. Herrera (2003), 'Health literacy in low-income Latino men and women receiving antiretroviral therapy in community-based treatment centers', *AIDS Patient Care and STDs*, 17 (6), pp. 283–298.
33 Friedland, R. B. (1998), 'Understanding health literacy: new estimates of the costs of inadequate health literacy', National Academy on an Ageing Society.
34 Kalichman, S. C. and D. Rompa (2000), 'Functional health literacy is associated with health status and health-related knowledge in people living with HIV-AIDS', *Journal of Acquired Immune Deficiency Syndromes*, 25 (4), pp. 337–344.
35 Baker, D. W., R. M. Parker, M. V. Williams, W. S. Clark and J. R. Nurss (1997), 'The relationship of patient reading ability to self-reported health and use of health services', *American Journal of Public Health*, 87 (6), pp. 1027–1030.
36 Gazmararian, J. A., D. W. Baker, R. M. Parker and D. G. Blazer (2000), 'A multivariate analysis of factors associated with depression: evaluating the role of health literacy as a potential contributor', *Archives of Internal Medicine*, 160 (21), pp. 3307–3314.
37 Baker, D. W., J. A. Gazmararian, J. Sudano, M. Patterson, R. M. Parker and M. V. Williams (2002), 'Health literacy and performance on the Mini-Mental State Examination', *Aging and Mental Health*, 6 (1), pp. 22–29.
38 Fortenberry, J. D., M. M. McFarlane, M. Hennessy, S. S. Bull, D. M. Grimley, J. St Lawrence, B. P. Stoner and N. VanDevanter (2001), 'Relation of health literacy to gonorrhoea related care', *Sexually Transmitted Infections*, 77 (3), pp. 206–211.
39 Baker, D. W., J. A. Gazmararian, M. V. Williams, T. L. Scott, R. M. Parker, D. C. Green, J. Ren and J. Peel (2002), 'Functional health literacy and the risk of hospital admission among Medicare managed care enrollees', *American Journal of Public Health*, 92 (8), pp. 1278–1283.
40 Guerra, C. E. and J. A. Shea (2003), 'Functional health literacy, comorbidity and health status', Abstract, *Journal of General Internal Medicine*, 18 (Supplement 1), p. 174.
41 Baker, D. W., R. M. Parker, M. V. Williams and W. S. Clark (1998), 'Health literacy and the risk of hospital admission', *Journal of General Internal Medicine*, 13 (12), pp. 791–798.
42 Weiss, B. D. and R. Palmer (2004), 'Relationship between health care costs and very low literacy skills in a medically needy and indigent Medicaid population', *Journal of the American Board of Family Practice*, 17 (1), pp. 44–47.
43 Howard, D. H. (2004), 'The relationship between health literacy and medical costs', in L. Nielsen-Bohlman, A. M. Panzer and D. A. Kindig

(eds.), Committee on Health Literacy, *Health Literacy: A Prescription To End Confusion*, Washington D. C.: National Academic Press.
44. Davis, T. C., R. Michielutte, E. N. Askov, M. V. Williams and B. D. Weiss (1998), 'Practical assessment of adult literacy in health care', *Health Education and Behavior*, 25, pp. 613–624.
45. Parker, R. M., D. W. Baker, M. V. Williams and J. R. Nurss (1995), 'The test of functional health literacy in adults: a new instrument for measuring patients' literacy skills', *Journal of General Internal Medicine*, 10 (10), pp. 537–541.
46. Davis, T. C., M. A. Crouch, S. W. Long, R. H. Jackson, P. Bates, R. B. George and L. E. Bairnsfather (1991), 'Rapid assessment of literacy levels of adult primary care patients', *Family Medicine*, 23 (6), pp. 433–435.
47. Kariya, T. (2001), *Kaisōka nippon to kyōiku kiki – fubyōdō sai seisan kara iyoku kakusa shakai (incentive divide) e* (Social stratification in Japan and education crises – from inequality reproduction to incentive divide), Tokyo: Yūshindō Kōbunsha.
48. Kariya, T. (1995), *Taishū kyōiku shakai no yukue – gakureki shugi to byōdō shinwa no sengo shi* (Trajectories of mass education society – post-war history of educational credentialism and equality-myth), Kyoto: Chūō Kōron Sha.
49. Tachibanaki, T., T. Saitō, T. Kariya and T. Satō (2004), *Fūin sareru fubyōdō* (Sealed Inequality), Tōyō Keizai Shinpō Sha.
50. Fukaya, T. (2001), I-bu, Kōreisha no shakai teki fubyōdō no sho sokumen, 2-shō, 'Kenkō to shinshin kinō' (Part I, Various aspects of social inequality among the elderly, Chapter 2, 'Health and psychosomatic functions'), in K. Hiraoka (ed.), *Kōrei ki to shakai teki fubyōdō* (Elderly Age and Social Inequality), Tokyo: University of Tokyo Press, pp. 29–50.
51. Matsuda, R., H. Hirai, K. Kondō, Y. Saitō and 'Kenkō no Fubyōdō' Kenkyū Kai ('Health Inequality' Study Group) (2005), 'Nippon no kōreisha – kaigo yobō ni muketa shakai ekigaku teki daikibo chōsa: kōreisha no hoken kōdō to tentō reki – shakai keizai teki chii to no sōkan (Elderly people in Japan – a large-scale social epidemiological survey for nursing-care-prevention: health care behaviour and history of falls of elderly people – correlation with socioeconomic status)', *Koshū Eisei* (Journal of Public Health Practice), 69, pp. 231–235.
52. Yoshii, K., K. Kondō, H. Hirai, R. Matsuda and Y. Saito (2005), 'Nippon no kōreisha – kaigo yobō ni muketa shakai ekigaku teki daikibo chōsa: kōreisha no shinshin kenkō no shakai keizai kakusa to chiiki kakusa no jittai (Elderly people in Japan – a large-scale social epidemiological survey for nursing-care-prevention: actual conditions of socioeconomic and regional disparities in psychosomatic health of the elderly)', *Koshū Eisei* (Journal of Public Health Practice), 69, pp. 145–148.
53. Hirai, H., K. Kondō, Y. Ichida and K. Suemori (2005), 'Nippon no kōreisha – kaigo yobō ni muketa shakai ekigaku teki daikibo chōsa: kōreisha no "tojikomori" (Elderly people in Japan – a large-scale social epidemiological survey for nursing-care-prevention: "social withdrawal" of elderly persons)', *Koshū Eisei* (Journal of Public Health Practice), 69, pp. 485–489.
54. Fujimura, M. (2001), I-bu, Kōreisha no shakai teki fubyōdō no sho sokumen, 1-shō, 'Shakai sanka, shakai teki nettowāku to jōhō akusesu'

(Part I, Various aspects of social inequality among the elderly, Chapter 1, 'Social participation, social network and information access'), in Kōichi Hiraoka (ed.), *Kōrei ki to shakai teki fubyōdō* (Elderly Age and Social Inequality), Tokyo: University of Tokyo Press, pp. 1–28.
55 Lemke, M., C. Calsyn, L. Lippman, L. Jocelyn, D. Kastberg, Y. Y. Liu, S. Roey, T. Williams, T. Kruger and G. Bairu (2001), *Outcome of learning: results from the 2000 program for international student assessment of 15-year-olds in reading, mathematics, and science literacy*, National Center for Education Statistics, (NCES 2000–115) Washington D. C. U.S. Government Printing Office.
56 Canada Ministry of Health (1999), *Communicating with Seniors: Advice, Techniques, and Tips*.
57 Gordon, M. M., R. Hampson, H. A. Capell and R. Madhok (2002), 'Illiteracy in rheumatoid arthritis patients as determined by the Rapid Estimate of Adult Literacy in Medicine (REALM) score', *Rheumatology* (Oxford), 41 (7), pp. 750–754.
58 Schillinger, D., J. Piette, K. Grumbach, F. Wang, C. Wilson, C. Daher, K. Leong-Grotz, C. Castro and A. B. Bindman (2003), 'Closing the loop: physician communication with diabetic patients who have low health literacy', *Archives of Internal Medicine*, 163 (1), pp. 83–90.
59 Kaufman, H., B. Skipper, L. Small, T. Terry and M. McGrew (2001), 'Effect of literacy on breast-feeding outcomes', *Southern Medical Journal*, 94 (3), pp. 293–296.

7 Gender and Health
Yuriko Doi

Introduction

In this chapter, I would like to present some concepts and theories on gender and health, and to confirm, through some social epidemiological studies, the scientific and social significance of this issue. I would also like to discuss the methodology and results of recent social epidemiological research, with some mention of its future prospects. Before taking up the main subject, I hope to deepen the understanding of gender and health by providing an overview of what 'gender' is, or more broadly, what 'sex' is, and what on earth is referred to by the term 'health' in this context.

Gender and sex

Social sex versus biological sex

A common concept of human sex would generally be 'biological sex', comprising males and females. As mentioned in more detail below, we often refer to sex using other terms in our society of human beings, namely, 'men' and 'women'. This concept of sex, as opposed to biological sex, can be called 'social sex' or 'gender' in the sense that it is determined by communities which have in turn been created by human beings. In either case, though, it seems that human beings are a species living in a dichotomous world consisting of the two sexes.

This dichotomous understanding of sex applies to the field of epidemiology as well. For instance, *A Dictionary of Epidemiology, Fourth Edition*[1] by John M. Last lists the term 'sex ratio'. This term is defined as 'The ratio of one sex to the other; usually defined as the ratio of males to females (or of the rates observed in males and females)' (p.167). This dictionary provides no definition or explanation of biological sex and only provides an explanation of 'social sex' or 'gender' as follows (p.75): 'In grammar, the term to designate a noun (person, animal, or object) as masculine, feminine or neuter. In parts of the English-speaking world, *gender* now signifies the totality of culturally-determined awareness, attitudes and beliefs about males and females and sometimes their sexual orientation. This usage may be politically correct ... [but] – for instance, in the headings of statistical tables – it is bewildering to readers whose first language has nouns that may carry any of three genders that are not necessarily related to the sex of the individual'.

Next, let me draw attention to the definitions of sex and gender adopted by the US National Institute of Health (NIH), the US National Academies' Institute of Medicine (IOM), and the World Health Organization (WHO).

In its *Agenda for Research on Women's Health for the 21st Century*[2], the NIH defines sex (males or females) as 'biologically defined differences' and gender (men or women) as 'differences that cannot merely be attributed to biological or physiological processes, but rather are almost always influenced by cultural, social and historical contexts' (pp.15–16). The IOM established the Committee on Understanding the Biology of Sex and Gender Differences comprising sixteen experts, including biologists, geneticists, medical scientists and others. The committee issued a report, *Exploring the biological contributions to human health: does sex matter?*[3], in which sex is defined as 'the classification of living things, generally as male or female according to their reproductive organs and functions assigned by chromosomal complement' and gender as 'a person's self-representation as male or female, or how that person is responded to by social institutions based on the individual's gender presentation. Gender is rooted in biology and shaped by environment and experience' (p.17).

Alternatively, in its technical book, *Gender and Health*[4], the WHO defines sex as 'genetic/physiological or biological characteristics of a person which indicate whether one is female or male' and gender as 'women's and men's roles and responsibilities that are socially determined. Gender is related to how we are perceived and expected to think and act as women and men because of the way society is organized, not because of our biological differences' (p.5).

The above definitions of 'sex' are virtually the same for the NIH, IOM and WHO. However, the three organisations define and use the term 'gender' in slightly different ways, in terms of their emphasis or focus. For instance, the IOM[3] defines sex and gender as 'biological sex' and 'social sex', respectively, and clearly distinguishes the two terms from each other in their usage. Meanwhile, the IOM mentions the difficulty of drawing a sharp line between sex and gender, taking the issue of gender identity as an example. In the field of psychology, gender identity refers to a person's understanding of his or her biological sex, including its psychological characteristics (the internalised sense of maleness or femaleness)[5]. Traditionally, the idea of gender identity has been based on the view that gender identity is determined by upbringing. The IOM mentions the view that androgen (male hormone) levels during the prenatal and early postnatal periods have a strong influence on the determination of gender identity and sex-specific behaviour. It points out that actually, there are many unknown mechanisms by which social and biological factors work together to form gender identity. On the other hand, the WHO focuses on gender roles and gender inequalities. It has taken up gender topics in the context of health issues, by developing health policies and implementing health sector reforms. The WHO has promoted the significance of gender equity and equality, particularly among researchers and policymakers[4].

Dichotomous and non-dichotomous sexes

As mentioned above, there is a concept of sex which regards human beings as a completely dimorphic species, whether in the sense of biological sex or social sex, comprising males and females or men and women, and categorises each and every person as one of two sexes. We live in this dichotomous world.

Alternative views argue that in fact there are not just two biological sexes for humans, but at least five: males, male pseudo-hermaphrodites, hermaphrodites, female pseudo-hermaphrodites, and females[6]. More importantly, biological characteristics in non-reproductive systems (e.g. voice and body hair, which are phenotypes affected by sex hormones) are rich in diversity. Some researchers support non-dichotomous concepts of sex as opposed to the firmly established dichotomous concept[6, 7].

Similarly, other researchers point out the difficulty of distinguishing between men and women using a clear dichotomy, such as masculinity versus femininity[8]. Let me ask you some simple questions here. Please respond 'Yes' if you think each of the following characteristics describes you, and 'No' if it doesn't: 1) inexpressive, 2) aggressive, 3) ambitious, 4) analytical, 5) assertive, 6) successful, 7) competitive, 8) forceful, 9) independent, 10) dominant, 11) strong personality, 12) athletic, 13) invulnerable, 14) emotional, 15) expressive, 16) compassionate, 17) childlike, 18) gentle, 19) loyal, 20) sensitive, 21) tender, 22) understanding, 23) yielding, 24) gullible, 25) refined, and 26) warm. How many 'Yes' answers did you have? The first thirteen items and the second thirteen items represent male and female gender stereotypes, respectively[8]. If you focus solely on your gender, completely irrespective of your biological sex, did you find that you are a 'man' (i.e. answered 'Yes' to all of the first half and 'No' to all of the second half of the questions), or a 'woman' (i.e. the exact opposite pattern of answers)? I expect that most of you found that you had some supposedly masculine and feminine characteristics (i.e. answered 'Yes' to some of the first half questions and to some of the second half questions).

Hence, human sex cannot always be divided simply into males and females, or men and women. For convenience, the community framework in which we live is based on the dichotomous concept of sex. Therefore, it is not hard to imagine that this dichotomous way of running our community may not always fit those of us who have non-dichotomous views of sex.

Factors determining social sex

I have thus far developed my argument based on the assumption that there exists social sex or gender (whether dichotomous or not). We seem to take the existence and definition of gender for granted because they agree with our actual feeling in real life. This is because we have seen in reality that ways of thinking and behaving which are expected of us, based on whether we are recognised as men or women, as well as the roles and responsibilities imposed on us as men or women, are determined by the community or organisation to which we belong. What then are the factors that determine gender? Before proceeding to a discussion of this issue, let me provide a brief summary of some definitions and views of sex from a legal perspective, with some mention of historical efforts in this field since World War II[9]. This is relevant because gender is generally determined by ourselves and our community, which in turn is run with a legal system as its basic framework.

After 1945 and World War II, the constitution of Japan came to guarantee equality of the sexes in suffrage, property rights and all other legal areas. This has meant that, under law, neither sex nor gender theoretically or formally exists (Table 7.1, column I). However, in reality, to this day laws have failed to get rid of sexual discrimination. In an international effort to overcome this problem, the 'Convention on the Elimination of All Forms of Discrimination against Women' (CEDAW) was adopted by the General Assembly of the United Nations in 1979 and came into force in 1981. This Convention regards any and all forms of different treatment by sex as discrimination in principle. The only permitted exception is different treatment based on pregnancy, childbirth and lactation, which are absolute sexual differences within the reproductive system; and this is accepted only for a limited period of time before and after childbirth. In former times (or even now), the idea of motherhood, that is, that women are the childbearing and childrearing gender, was widespread in society. The Convention declares that there are no sex differences in childrearing and, therefore, does not allow the exception to be applied to childrearing. Moreover, the Convention regards maternity protection measures (such as prohibition of late-night or holiday work, and restrictions on engaging in hazardous activities), which used to be applicable to women only, as discrimination against women. It also adopts the stance that any forms of different treatment based on physical characteristics that are related to non-reproductive sex differences are unacceptable (Table 7.1, column II). Japan ratified this convention in 1985, and it forms the basis of Japan's current gender equality policy.

Let us now return to the question of what factors determine gender. The essential determinants of gender are discrimination of treatment based on sex within all areas of a community. The international community reached agreement on this, and in 1980, steered towards complete elimination of discrimination against women. The reason why the target was women is because most of those who had suffered systemic sexual discrimination in their communities had historically been women.

This epoch-making movement in the global community greatly influenced the field of health sciences. In the traditional biomedical field, sex meant biological sex only (Table 7.1, column III). To this, the movement added social sex, a completely different concept (Table 7.1, column IV). The new concept seems to have been quite controversial at first, but after a quarter of a century, the term and concept of gender has generally become accepted in the field of health sciences.

Let me now provide a brief summary of factors determining gender. The essential determinants of biological sex are the sex chromosomes. The place of their manifestation is mainly in the reproductive organs; as well, there are physical attributes and functions affected by the sex chromosomes. At the same time, the

Table 7.1: Differences in treatment by sex

	I	II	III	IV
Biological sex				
Reproductive system	–	+	+	+
Non-reproductive systems	–	–	+	+
Social sex	–	–	–	+

Notes.

I: There are no absolute or relative biological sexual differences (i.e. differences in the reproductive system or non-reproductive systems, respectively) and no sexual differences in social characteristics.

II: There are absolute biological sexual differences (i.e. differences in the reproductive system) only.

III: There are absolute and relative biological sexual differences (i.e. differences in the reproductive system and non-reproductive systems, respectively) only.

IV: There are absolute and relative biological sexual differences (i.e. differences in the reproductive system or non-reproductive systems, respectively) and sexual differences in social characteristics.

essential determinants of gender are acts of discrimination by sex in ways of thinking and behaving that are expected of us, and in the roles and responsibilities that are imposed on us because of our sex. The main areas where this is apparent are 1) in households, 2) in workplaces, 3) in political and economic organisations, and 4) in health-care settings. Its respective basic manifestations in these fields would include 1) housework, childrearing and nursing care; 2) employment, wages and occupational positions; 3) participation in politics (voting and eligibility for election) and distribution of resources (assets and income); and 4) access to health-care services[10–12]. One basic difference between biological sex and social sex is that the latter can be changed by manipulating or intervening in the determining factors.

Social sex or gender as a health outcome

Are there any sexual differences in health? If so, do they arise from biological differences or social ones, or both? And what are the mechanisms by which they cause health differences? In order to answer these questions, researchers in the traditional biomedical field have studied how biological sex is involved in people's physical and mental health (the biomedical paradigm, Figure 7.1). In this context, biological sex has been treated mainly as a confounder

Figure 7.1: Three paradigms of biological and social sex, and health

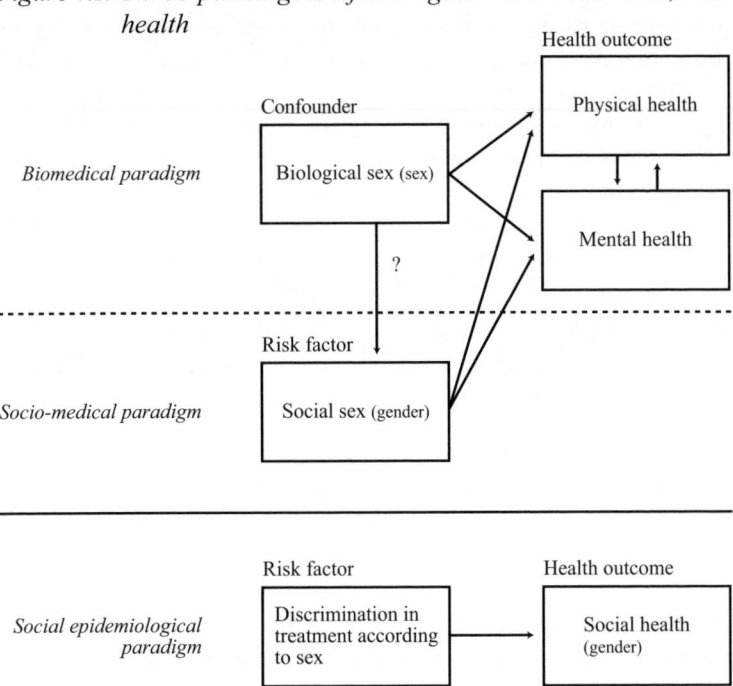

Note: For simplification, other related factors have been omitted.

as it cannot usually be changed. On the other hand, gender, as a socially-determined trait, can be changed. This has led in recent years to studies emerging in the field of social medicine which treat gender as a risk factor and discuss how it is involved in physical and mental health[12]. Furthermore, the need has been recognized for more integrated models which consider both sex and gender at the same time[13], and for interdisciplinary research on this issue (the socio-medical paradigm, Figure 7.1).

In its constitution, the WHO defines health as not only being free from disease but also having physical, psychological and social well-being[14]. With this definition in mind, we find that the essence of gender, as a social issue, may be considered a deviation from social well-being. The existence of gender itself can represent a poor health outcome. While the ratification of conventions and institution of systems for eliminating sexual discrimination has progressed, our societies have not been able to fully catch up with this movement in reality. In other words, this gap, created by the failure to catch up, represents the poor social health or social well-being caused by sexual discrimination. How we should bridge this gap is likely to become a key point in developing research and measures concerning gender and health in the future. To do so, I believe the field of health sciences will need to develop a paradigm that is different from the conventional one on gender and health. What we will need is a paradigm which treats gender itself as a health outcome, representing poor social well-being, and which regards sex discrimination, which is the determining factor of gender, as a risk factor (the social epidemiological paradigm, Figure 7.1). In this context, biological sex itself is not to be regarded as a health outcome, and this seems to be another basic difference between gender and biological sex.

Sex or gender differences in sleep

Certain epidemiological studies on sleep will be presented and discussed from a socio-medical viewpoint of sex or gender differences in the first half of this section. That should distinguish what has been evident concerning this issue from what has not. In the second half, gender differences observed in our society will be discussed through the lens of sleep research.

Differences based on epidemiological research in Japan

Sleep and related problems in the general adult population of Japan

In 1997, a nationwide survey on sleep and health was conducted on a representative sample of Japanese adults, aged 20 years and over, to estimate the prevalence of insomnia and regular use of hypnotic medication, and to identify high risk groups[15]. The subjects were 2,800 adult males and females, randomly selected from all over Japan. An anonymous self-administered questionnaire on sleep and health was sent to and collected from these subjects by mail (response rate: 67.5%). In this survey, the Pittsburgh Sleep Quality Index (PSQI) was used to assess the subjects' sleep. 'Difficulty initiating sleep' (DIS) was defined as the inability to fall asleep within 30 minutes at a frequency of at least three times weekly in the past month; 'difficulty in maintaining sleep' (DMS) was defined as awakening during the night or in the early morning at the same frequency as above; and 'insomnia' was defined as experiencing the symptoms of either DIS or DMS at the same frequency as above.

Figure 7.2: Prevalence of insomnia

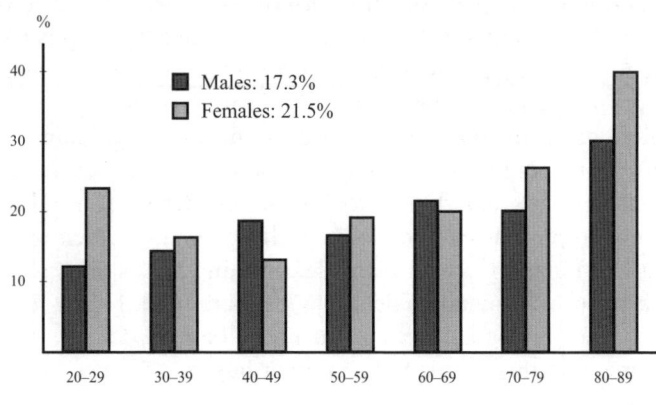

Note: Effects of age were seen in both sexes. p < 0.05; no sex differences.
Source: adapted from Doi, et al (2000)[15].

As for hypnotic medication use (HMU), 'regular use' was defined as use of such medication to fall asleep at the same frequency as above. In addition, 'poor subjective sleep quality' was defined as self-reported occurrence of poor sleep quality at the same frequency as above in the past month. The analysis was made for 1,871 subjects (920 males and 951 females), and excluded those who responded as sex 'unknown'. The prevalence was calculated for each sex and each age group based on the above definitions. In addition, the age-adjusted prevalence was estimated for each sex, based on the age distribution of data from the 1995 national census. Furthermore, statistical tests were conducted to detect the effects of age and sex differences.

The prevalence of insomnia (95% confidence interval) was 17.3% (14.6–20.2%) and 21.5% (18.8–24.3%) for males and females, respectively. In both sexes, the prevalence of insomnia tended to increase with age (p<0.05). In particular, the prevalence of insomnia in males and females aged 80 and over was as high as 30.5% and 40.3%, respectively (Figure 7.2). No statistical significance in sex differences was found for insomnia. Interesting results were revealed when the two symptoms of DIS and DMS were analysed separately. For DIS, as shown in Figure 7.3, females showed a significantly higher prevalence than males: 12.6% (10.4–14.8%) and 8.6% (5.6–10.6%), respectively. The effects of age were found

Figure 7.3: Prevalence of difficulty initiating sleep

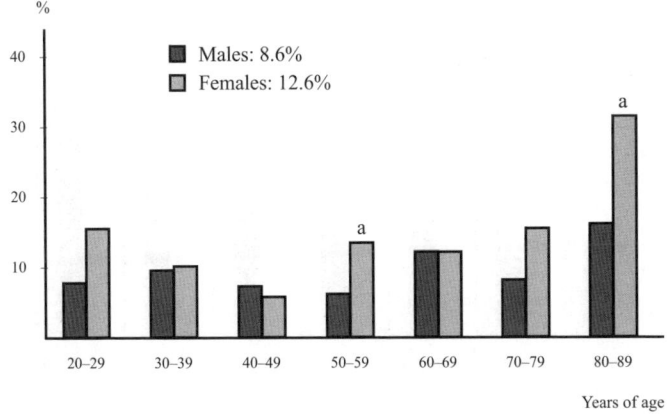

Notes: Effects of age were seen in females only. $p < 0.05$.
a: sex difference ($p < 0.05$).
Source: adapted from Doi, et al (2000)[15].

among females only, with females in their fifties and eighties showing remarkably high prevalence ($p<0.05$). For DMS, the prevalence figures for males and females were 12.9% (10.6–15.3%) and 16.2% (13.8–18.6%), respectively. The effects of age were seen in both sexes ($p<0.05$). The prevalence of DMS in females was higher than in males but only for subjects in their twenties ($p<0.05$) (Figure 7.4).

Similar results have been reported in other surveys[16]. In 1997, an epidemiological survey by means of interviews was conducted to examine the association between insomnia and lifestyles and health among 4,000 Japanese adults aged 20 years and over who were randomly selected largely from urban areas (response rate: 75.8%). In this survey, 'insomnia' was defined as always or often experiencing at least one symptom of difficulty initiating sleep (DIS), night awakening and early morning awakening. The prevalence of insomnia based on the above definition was 22.3% (20.1–24.5%) and 20.5% (18.4–22.6%) for males and females, respectively, showing no sex difference. The prevalence for subjects aged 60 years and over was about double that of the subjects between ages 20 and 39. For DIS, the overall prevalence rates for both sexes were estimated at 8.3% (7.3–9.4%). The prevalence was about 1.4 times higher for females than males, but no effects of age were found. For 'night

Figure 7.4: Prevalence of difficulty maintaining sleep

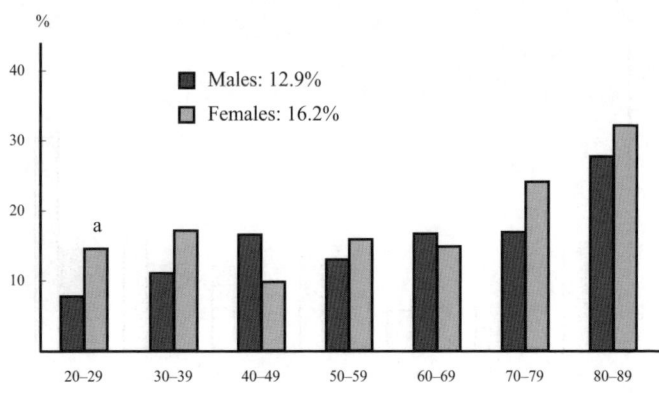

Notes: Effects of age were seen in both sexes. p < 0.05.
a: sex difference (p < 0.05).
Source: adapted from Doi, et al (2000)[15].

awakening' and 'early morning awakening', the overall prevalence rates for both sexes were 15.0% (13.6–16.3%) and 8.0 (7.0–9.0%), respectively. The effects of age were seen in both symptoms of night awakening and early morning awakening (the prevalence was significantly higher – 2.4 and 3.0 times, respectively – for subjects aged 60 and over, than for those aged between 20 and 39), but no differences between sexes were found.

Figure 7.5 shows the prevalence of medication use for sleep at least three times weekly during the past month[15]. The prevalence is likely to represent the proportion of subjects who chronically used hypnotic medication rather than those who used it temporarily. The age-adjusted prevalence rates of HMU were 3.5% (2.3–3.7%) and 5.4% (4.1–6.8%) for males and females, respectively. For each sex, the prevalence of HMU tended to increase with age (p < 0.05). In particular, females aged 80 and over had a remarkably high prevalence (over 20%). In terms of sex differences, the prevalence of HMU was significantly higher among females than males aged 80 and over and those in their fifties (p < 0.05). This is similar to the pattern seen in the prevalence of DIS shown in Figure 7.3. The differences between the pattern of prevalence rates seen in HMU and DIS are that as a matter of course, the former is lower than the latter. For females in their fifties and those aged 80 and over,

Figure 7.5: Prevalence of hypnotic medication use

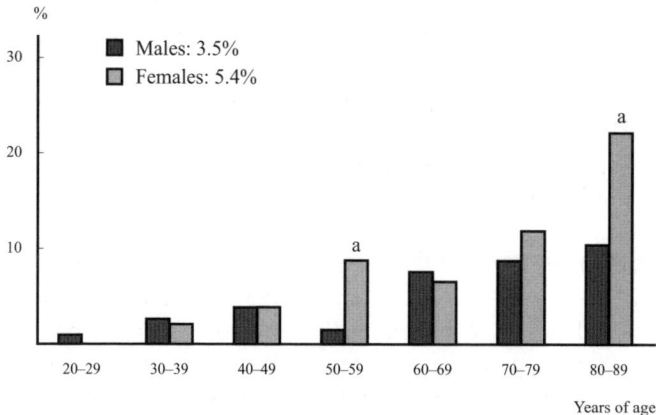

Notes: Effects of age were seen in both sexes. p < 0.05.
a: Sex difference (p < 0.05).
Source: adapted from Doi, et al (2000)[15].

it was suggested that they tended to have trouble getting to sleep and were, compared to other sex-age groups, more likely to use hypnotic medication on a regular basis to induce sleep. A relatively high proportion of females in their twenties had DIS, while they showed a very low prevalence of HMU.

Sleep and related problems in the working population of Japan
Recent years have seen more attention being paid to the sleep and related problems of Japanese workers[17]. However, few epidemiological studies have focused on gender differences in workers' sleep and related problems. In fact, only a small number of women work full-time for companies in Japan, which makes it impossible to collect a sufficient sample size of female workers for analysing gender differences. Also as a result, those who happen to be included among the subjects of a survey would be either excluded from any analysis or analysed together with men. In nine out of the thirteen Japanese epidemiological studies on the sleep of workers, the subjects comprised male workers only[17].

In 1999 and 2000, epidemiological research on sleep and health was conducted on about 6,000 workers between the ages of 20 and 59 years who worked for companies located in the Tokyo metropolitan area (response rates: 91.0% and 85.9% for 1999 and 2000, respectively). It attempted to comprehensively assess subjective sleep, including insomnia, poor sleep quality and excessive daytime sleepiness in 4,868 workers (4,003 men and 865 women) excluding shift workers. The PSQI was used as the assessment measure. 'Poor sleep quality' was defined as scoring six points or more on the PSQI. The prevalence of 'poor sleep quality' was calculated for each gender-age group[18]. The results showed that the prevalence was significantly higher for the subjects of this survey (Figure 7.7) than general adults (Figure 7.6) in all gender-age groups, except women in their twenties; the prevalence ranged between 32.6% and 43.9% among men, and between 41.8% and 44.6% for women[18,19]. With advancing age, the prevalence decreased in men and increased in women. For workers in their fifties, women had poorer sleep quality than men, which was consistent with the previous study for general adult populations. Workers with poor sleep quality were more likely to suffer subjective poor health (approx. 5 times more), take sick leave (approx. 2 times more), and have problems in occupational activities or personal relationships (each, approx. 2.5 times more). They were also more likely to have accidents (approx. 2 times more), although a significant difference was not detected due to the small number of accidents involved. Factors associated with poor sleep quality included stress, job dissatisfaction, hypertension, poor bedroom environment, younger age and being single.

For workers, 'excessive daytime sleepiness' (EDS) may cause serious problems in terms of work efficiency and safety. The prevalence of EDS was calculated for the same research subjects as above, by using the Epworth Sleepiness Scale, which measures subjective daytime sleepiness [20]. The prevalence rates were 7.2% and 13.3% for men and women, respectively; the latter was significantly higher than the former. Hours of sleep were significantly fewer for women than for men; 65.3% and 76.5% of men and women, respectively, had less than seven hours of sleep, and 22.7% and 31.7% of men and women, respectively, had less than six hours of sleep. The percentage of participants who reported subjective poor sleep was significantly higher for women (53.4%) than men (40.3%). Men (57.9%) had a slightly higher rate of affirmative answers to having an irregular bedtime and wakeup time than women (54.2%). While men (17.8%) had considerable day-to-day variations in bedtime and wakeup time, women (44.0%) had variations in bedtime and wakeup time between weekdays and weekends. Each of these three factors (hours of sleep, quality of sleep, and sleep-wake rhythm) was significantly associated with

Figure 7.6 Prevalence of poor sleep quality (among the general population)

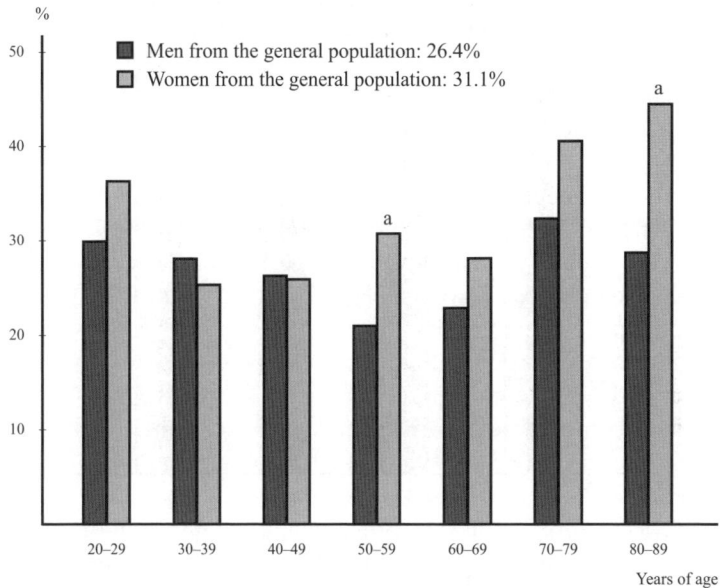

Notes: Effects of age were seen in both sexes. p<0.05
a: Gender difference.
Source: adapted from Doi, et al (2001)[18].

EDS in both men and women. Interestingly, marital status and family status had completely different effects on EDS for men and women. For women, those who lived with family members who required parenting or nursing care were more likely to report EDS. For men, on the other hand, they were less likely to report EDS under the same circumstances as women. In addition, married men were less likely to report EDS. EDS had a significant association with depressed moods in both men and women.

Gender differences in society as seen through sleep research

The results described above suggest that there are likely to be sex or gender differences for sleep and related problems, and in coping behaviours, such as taking hypnotic medication, and that the differences are likely to exist at different stages of a life-course. Some research issues remain to be unravelled in the studies

Figure 7.7: Prevalence of poor sleep quality (among workers)

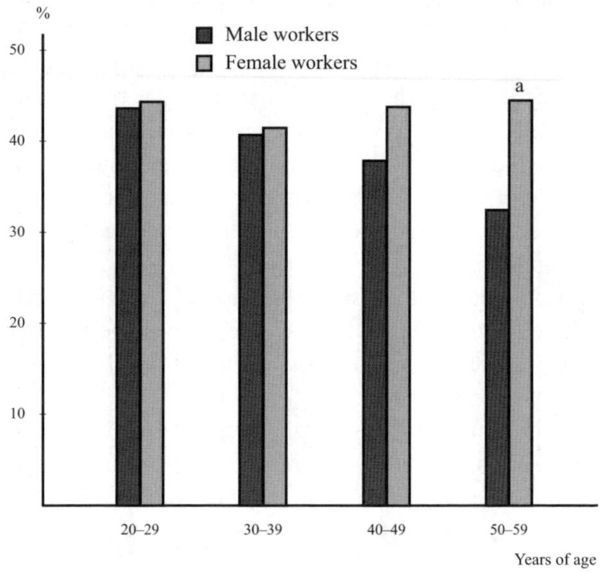

[Bar chart showing prevalence (%) of poor sleep quality by age group (20–29, 30–39, 40–49, 50–59) for male and female workers. Male workers: ~44, ~41, ~38, ~33. Female workers: ~44, ~42, ~44, ~45. The 50–59 group shows a gender difference marked "a".]

Notes: Effects of age were seen in both sexes. p < 0.05.
a: Gender difference
Source: adapted from Doi, Minowa & Tango (2003)[19].

described above: whether the differences in sleep and related problems arise from biological or social sex differences or both; and if the latter is the case, to what degree or extent does each contribute to generating the differences, and how do the mechanisms work?

Gender differences in our society appear through the lens of sleep research, when looking at research results from the viewpoint of gender. For instance, a high prevalence of DMS for women in their twenties may reflect the interruption of sleep due to caring for their children at night. A high prevalence of DIS and poor sleep quality for women in their fifties may be associated with the biological effects of menopause as well as the psychosocial crisis stemming from gender roles unique to women at this critical age. A high prevalence of DIS and poor sleep quality for elderly women may result from not only their own illnesses but also the burden of caring for their ailing spouses (elder-to-elder nursing care). Regarding hypnotic medication, the high prevalence of use among middle-aged and elderly women may reflect a gender-free benefit of the universal health care system, under which their access to medical institutions was not restricted because of their female gender. In this regard, it is necessary to consider the reason, from the viewpoint of gender, why a small number of women in their twenties had been prescribed hypnotic medication despite a high prevalence of DIS. Another point worth noting is that for full-time workers, the effects of having spouses and families on men and women were the opposite. While having spouses and families was associated with good sleep and higher daytime arousal levels in men, it was associated with sacrificing sleep and excessive daytime sleepiness in women.

Epidemiological studies have shown that sleep is significantly associated with health and safety (subjective well-being, depressed moods, sick leave and accidents), as well as 'quality of life' and productivity (personal relationships and work). This has made us realize the importance of good sleep for our well-being and lives. Currently in the biomedical field, research has been steadily progressing towards endorsing the value of good sleep (e.g. clinical research on pharmacotherapy, cognitive behavioural therapy and phototherapy, and basic research on sleep-wake mechanisms). What if, though, the differences of social sex or gender are involved in this issue as a factor affecting sleep? This needs a new research project which takes biological sex as well as social sex into consideration. Sex-specific and/or gender-specific medicines are required for therapy and intervention from the viewpoints of sex and gender differences.

Future prospects

Finally, I would like to make some comments and suggestions on the issue of gender and health with some mention of its future prospects.

As mentioned above, in its effort to eliminate sexual discrimination, Japan joined the CEDAW of the United Nations in 1985, and this was followed by the promulgation and enforcement of the Basic Law for a Gender-Equal Society in 1999. Under this law, Japan has taken active improvement measures based on the following five basic principles: (i) respect for the human rights of men and women (Article 3), (ii) consideration of social systems or practices (Article 4), (iii) joint participation in planning and decision-making policies, etc (Article 5), (iv) compatibility of activities in family life and other activities (Article 6), (v) international cooperation (Article 7). For instance, the Basic Plan for Gender Equality was adopted by the Cabinet in 2000.

The Basic Plan lists eleven key goals. To achieve these goals by 2010, the local governments of Japan have set their own numerical targets and increased their efforts that take local characteristics into account. Thus, the momentum for approaches to gender in Japan has been based on the respect for, and the protection of, human rights – the core of the gender issue. This seems to have resulted in a situation where the understanding that gender itself as a health issue has been missing, even in the field of health sciences. The existence of gender itself represents poor social health or well-being, resulting from discriminatory treatment based on sex. Shouldn't we stop treating the gender issue as a peripheral problem in the field of health science, and instead, regard it as one of the more central issues?

There are three promising approaches within social epidemiological research for resolving the gender issue in the field of health sciences. The first is community-based intervention studies (the social epidemiological paradigm). For instance, a program which has been developed to change the sense of gender roles in a workplace or community could be randomly introduced to two groups: an intervention group and a control group. The study could test a hypothesis and evaluate the intervention by analysing whether any differences are found between the two groups in terms of gender roles or empowerment. The second is analytical epidemiological studies focusing on the elucidation of mechanisms (the socio-medical paradigm). A human being is not divided into two parts – his/her social sex and biological sex. These two aspects of sex are intricately linked, not only with each other but with other factors as well, and with this, each person lives in his/her ecosystem called society (Figure 7.8)[21, 22]. Some describe this as 'the web of causation'[23] in which factors are linked with each other like a cobweb. Researchers' desire to unravel this web of causation stems from a purely scientific motive: to know more about human beings. Results from research are likely to lead to the development and implementation of more effective intervention. The third approach is validation studies on equal employment opportunities for both sexes in an effort to eliminate gender differences (the social epidemiological paradigm and socio-medical paradigm). In accordance with the CEDAW, the prohibition of women doing late-night and holiday work, and the restriction on women doing hazardous activities were abolished. This may certainly be reasonable in terms of equality of the sexes and ensuring some choice with respect to employment. However, in light of the present situation in Japan, where the number of

Figure 7.8: Concept of health and aging

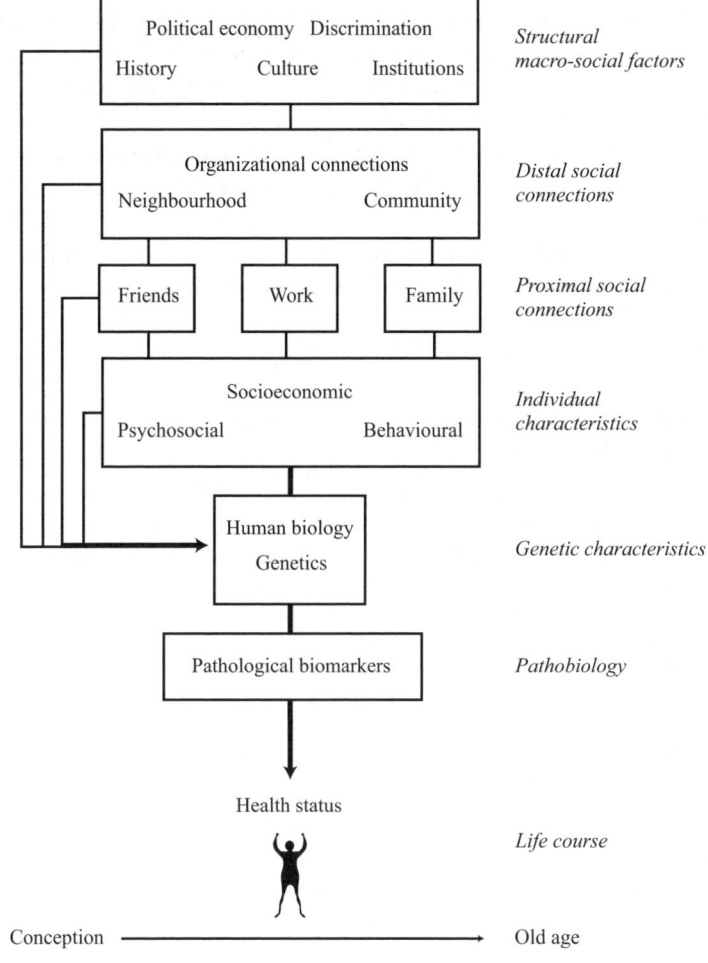

Source: Lynch (2000)[21]. Reproduced with kind permission from Dr. J. Rayner, Editor, *Australasian Epidemiologist*, and Dr. J. Lynch.

deaths from overwork has been increasing since 1988, a question arises as to whether women should have to adapt to men's work practices (e.g. regular overwork) in order to work on equal terms. So far, most deaths from overwork have occurred among men; hence, should the number of deaths from overwork among women be allowed to increase to the male level? It seems necessary then to validate the effect of equal employment opportunities for both sexes on gender equality or inequality from the viewpoint of health.

As the 'discovery' of gender and the appeal of gender issues to society have been largely attributed to feminists, the issue of gender and health has mostly been dealt with from the stance of women. Recent years have seen some studies, reports and suggestions from the viewpoint of men[8, 24, 25]. These have helped people become more aware of the importance of health differences related to gender. The ultimate goal of the issue on gender and health would be the pursuit of humanity and human nature beyond the dichotomy of masculinity versus femininity or fatherhood versus motherhood.

Literature

1. Last, J. M. (2001), *A Dictionary of Epidemiology, Fourth Edition*, Oxford: Oxford University Press, p. 75.
2. Fishman, J. R., J. G. Wick and B. A. Koenig (1999), 'The use of "sex" and "gender" to define and characterize meaningful differences between men and women', in U.S. Department of Health and Human Services, Public Health Services, National Institute of Health, *Agenda for research on women's health for the 21st century. A Report of the Task Force on the NIH Women's Health Research Agenda for the 21st Century, Volume 2* (NIH Publication No. 99–4386), Bethesda (MD): NIH, pp. 15–22.
3. Weizemann, T. M. and M.-L. Pardue (eds) (2001), *Exploring the biological contributions to human health: does sex matter?*, Washington DC: National Academy Press.
4. World Health Organization (1998), *Gender and Health: a Technical Paper*, Geneva: World Health Organization.
5. Notman, M. T. and C. C. Nadelson (1995), 'Gender, development, and psychopathology', in M. V. Seeman (ed), *Gender and Psychopathology*, Washington DC: American Psychiatric Press, Inc., pp. 1–16.
6. Fausto-Sterling, A. (1993), 'The five sexes', *The Sciences*, March/April, pp. 20–25.
7. Fausto-Sterling, A. (2000), 'The five sexes, revised', *The Sciences*, July/August, pp. 19–23.
8. Moynihan, C. (2000), 'Theories in health care and research: theories of masculinity', *British Medical Journal*, 317, pp. 1072–1075.
9. Yokota, K. (1997), 'Sei-sabetsu to byōdō gensoku (Sex discrimination and the equality principle)', in *Gendai no hō 11: jendā to hō* (Modern Law, vol. 11: Gender and Law), Tokyo: Iwanami Shoten, pp. 71–100 (in Japanese).
10. Moss, N. E. (2002), 'Gender equity and socioeconomic inequality: a framework for the patterning of women's health', *Social Science & Medicine*, 54, pp. 649–661.
11. Krieger, N. (2003), 'Gender, sexes and health: what are the connections – and why does it matter?', *International Journal of Epidemiology*, 32, pp. 652–657.

12 Kawachi, I., B. P. Kennedy, V. Gupta and D. Prothrow-Stith (1999), 'Women's status and the health of women and men: a review from the States', *Social Science & Medicine*, 48, pp. 21–32.
13 Bird, C. E. and P. P. Rieker (1999), 'Gender matters: an integrated model for understanding men's and women's health', *Social Science & Medicine*, 48, pp. 745–755.
14 World Health Organization (1948), *Constitution in Basic Documents*, Geneva: World Health Organization.
15 Doi, Y., M. Minowa, M. Ōkawa and M. Uchiyama (2000), 'Prevalence of sleep disturbance and hypnotic medication use in relation to socio-demographic factors in the general Japanese adult population', *Journal of Epidemiology*, 10, pp. 79–86.
16 Kim, K., M. Uchiyama, M. Ōkawa, X. Liu and R. Ogihara (2000), 'An epidemiological study of insomnia among the Japanese general population', *Sleep*, 23, pp. 1–7.
17 Doi, Y. (2005), 'An epidemiologic review on occupational sleep research among Japanese workers', *Industrial Health*, 43, pp. 3–10.
18 Doi, Y., M. Minowa, M. Uchiyama and M. Ōkawa (2001), 'Subjective sleep quality and sleep problems in the general Japanese adult population', *Psychiatry and Clinical Neurosciences*, 55, pp. 213–215.
19 Doi, Y., M. Minowa and T. Tango (2003), 'Impact and correlates of poor sleep quality in Japanese white-collar employees', *Sleep*, 26, pp. 467–471.
20 Doi, Y. and M. Minowa (2002), 'Gender difference in excessive daytime sleepiness among Japanese workers', *Social Science & Medicine*, 56, pp. 883–894.
21 Lynch, J. W. (2000), 'Social epidemiology: some observations on the past, present and future', *Australasian Epidemiologist*, 7, pp. 7–15.
22 Bartley, M., A. Sacker, I. Schoon and K. Hunt (2002), 'Social and economic trajectories and women's health', in D. Kuh and R. Hardy (eds), *A Life Course Approach to Women's Health*, Oxford: Oxford University Press, pp. 233–254.
23 Krieger, N. (1994), 'Epidemiology and the web of causation: has anyone seen the spider?', *Social Science & Medicine*, 39, pp. 887–903.
24 Kraemer, S. (2000), 'The fragile male', *British Medical Journal*, 321, pp. 1609–1613.
25 Doyal, L. (2001), 'Sex, gender and health: the need for a new approach', *British Medical Journal*, 323, pp. 1061–1063.

8 Culture and Health
Noboru Iwata

What is culture?

Defining culture

In anthropology, sociology and related disciplines, there have been arguments about how to understand culture for a very long time. Examples of classical definitions of culture include: 'Culture or civilization, taken in its wide ethnographic sense, is that complex whole which includes knowledge, belief, art, morals, law, custom, and any other capabilities and habits acquired by man as a member of society'[1]; and 'Culture consists of patterns, explicit or implicit, of and for behaviour acquired and transmitted by symbols constituting the distinctive achievement of human groups, including their embodiments in artifacts'[2].

One modern definition of culture is that issued by UNESCO in 2002: 'Culture should be regarded as the set of distinctive spiritual, material, intellectual and emotional features of society or a social group, and that it encompasses, in addition to art and literature, lifestyles, ways of living together, value systems, traditions and beliefs'[3]. Cultures are complex, hierarchical systems that comprise an extremely wide range of practices and behaviour patterns; these range from people's everyday life practices, involving housing, food and clothing, to social structures, such as public entertainment, morals, religion, politics and economics.

The concept of culture is applied to a human population above a certain size (i.e. a community). A geographical area sharing the same cultural style is called a 'cultural area'. A person who is born in a certain cultural area is taught and learns the local culture through a process of socialisation during his/her development. A particular culture adapts around life in a community, and education serves to provide community members, as members of that cultural area, with necessary knowledge. Spoken and written language is used for communication in this process of learning.

A linguistic system reflects the mental processes of people living in the cultural area in which the linguistic system is contained. A particular linguistic system covers all the basic elements of local lifestyles, such as personal relationships, values, norms, beliefs and attitudes. In this sense, language is not just a component of culture but plays a major role as a medium for maintaining the culture. This understanding is reflected in an attempt to assess the levels of acceptance by immigrants and their descendants of the host country's culture, based on their levels of understanding and frequency of use of the language of their new homeland[4].

Cultural awareness in epidemiology and socio-medical research

In traditional socio-medical research, cultural factors have not been dealt with directly as explanatory variables. Rather, cultural factors have been excluded from analysis because they can be considerably ambiguous and may hinder more traditional scientific approaches.

Epidemiological studies in multi-racial/ethnic countries like the USA have almost always included racial/ethnic variables in their analysis. While race is a more biological term which implies common physical characteristics, ethnicity is more of a cultural/ psychological term which implies common social affiliation[5]. However, previous studies have failed to distinguish between race and ethnicity and have used them simply as confounding factors to be controlled in statistical analysis[6]. This is because in most of these studies, the primary objective was to detect potential associations between risk factors and health indices that are common to all people irrespective of race or ethnicity. Cultural factors have been regarded as elements of bias in attempts to detect true associations.

On the other hand, with international comparisons of health indices, researchers have often discussed social (cultural) differences which may affect health indices. These studies have been based on a simplified model which assumes that a country is the same as a cultural area. Thus, they have failed to allow for some specific cultural variables, and have remained on the same level as studies focusing on comparisons between different races or ethnic groups[7].

In this chapter, I focus on physical health status, which has been a target of many previous epidemiological studies, and discuss cultural factors that affect physical health status. Unfortunately, only a small number of studies have thus far demonstrated an association between physical health status and aspects of culture. This shows the difficulty of scientifically demonstrating the direct association between culture and health, and so please note that the discussion in this chapter simply represents my own personal views.

Understanding culture within social epidemiology

Hierarchical understanding of culture

Different geographical areas, different populations and different eras have resulted in different cultures. The relationship between culture and an individual living in that culture is similar to the figure-ground relationship in Gestalt psychology. Specifically, we could say that an individual is located in the foreground and the culture he/she lives in is the backdrop. Therefore, if we focus on the individual level, it can be difficult to observe the culture at the same time[5].

It is practically impossible to identify all of the components of culture listed in the UNESCO definition[3]. However, if we look at some lifestyle guidelines describing the pathogenesis, treatment and prevention (of recurrences) of non-infectious chronic diseases, which constitute the main types of disease at the present time, we realise that there are a number of significant risk factors and aggravating factors (or preventive and improvement factors) lurking in a culture. Specifically, these factors include values, norms, behaviour patterns and lifestyles (and the learning and diffusion of these) that are unique to a certain culture.

Values are beliefs commonly shared by members of the community, or group norms internalised by an individual. By learning these values, a member of the community comes to understand and maintain the behavioural rules of the broad community. In this sense, its system of values seems to constitute the core components of a culture.

Incidentally, one characteristic of approaches to social epidemiology research is the use of multilevel analysis. This approach allows analysis which makes good use of a special characteristic of the data (a hierarchical structure), and reveals potential effects of explanatory variables on each hierarchical level, and of interactions between different levels of health indicators (objective variables) (see Chapter 10). When we discuss culture as a factor affecting health problems of individuals and the population, we realise that the components of culture are very hierarchical. For the purposes of this discussion, I have experimented with classifying cultural factors

Figure 8.1: Hierarchical understanding of culture

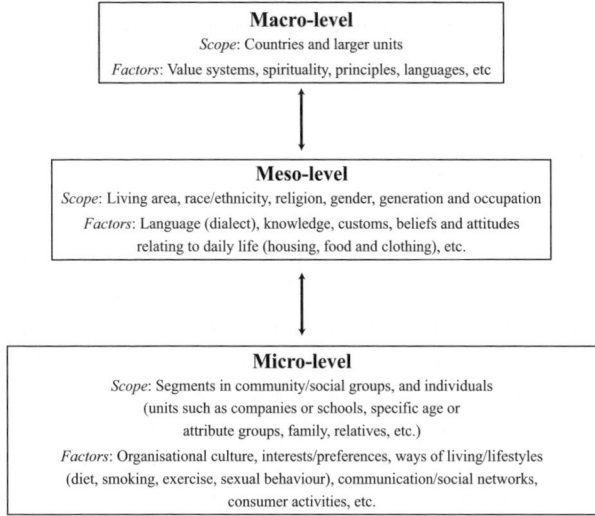

into three levels, macro-, meso- and micro- (Figure 8.1), when discussing them as variables affecting health in social epidemiology.

Macro-level

The macro-level refers to cultural differences between different countries or larger units. Factors at this level include the system of values, mental characteristics, beliefs and language.

Geert Hofstede[8] conducted the same values survey of IBM employees in fifty countries worldwide and produced the following five dimensions: individualism-collectivism, power/distance, uncertainty avoidance, short-term/long-term orientation, and femininity-masculinity. The most widely known of these is the individualism-collectivism dimension which shows the degree to which a person behaves, thinks and exists as an individual or as a member of a community[9].

On the other hand, Michael H. Bond[10] conducted a questionnaire survey of university students in twenty-one countries worldwide and extracted two value dimensions: social integration-cultural inwardness, and reputation-social morality. Social integration is a belief that values patience and harmony with others, and emphasises self-control, non-competition, trust and persistence. Cultural inwardness includes finding value in the protection of tradition, a sense of cultural superiority, maintenance of socially-established ceremonies, et cetera. The reputation-social morality dimension can be described as an axis along which the degree to which one 'makes him/herself look better' is measured, as compared to the degree to which one 'behaves well'.

Meso-level

The meso-level refers to cultural differences that exist between different communities or social groups, which are, in turn, members of the same cultural area at the macro-level (which is a country, in most cases). In this context, 'communities' or 'social groups' refer to units of living areas determined by geographical distribution; ethnic or religious groups; groups based on gender, generation or occupation; and other units which are independent of geographical distribution. These constitute cultures at the meso-level, as subsets within a country (i.e. within a macro-level cultural area).

Typical examples of cultural factors at the meso-level include language (dialect), knowledge and customs relating to everyday life, such as housing, food and clothing, and beliefs and attitudes relating to such knowledge and customs. Social class and social capital, which are detailed in Chapters 3 and 9, respectively, are additional examples of meso-level cultural factors. However, if you think of Spanish-speaking South American countries (not Brazil), it may be awkward to regard language as a meso-level cultural factor. Nonetheless, in a multilingual, multiracial country, language and other meso-level cultural factors are two sides of the same coin. Psychiatric studies on immigrant populations have frequently used language as an indicator of the levels of acceptance of the host country's culture[4]. This is because the levels so measured correspond with the degrees to which the subculture (a meso-level cultural factor) is maintained against the main culture in the macro-level cultural area.

Micro-level

The micro-level refers to cultural factors that vary within different segments or subdivisions of the communities and social groups constituting the meso-level culture. Hence, micro-level cultural factors are subdivisions of the meso-level cultural factors. Examples of micro-level cultural factors include organisational cultures seen in companies and schools, customs existing in families or extended family units, and interests, preferences and behaviour patterns seen within age or attribute groups. Additional examples are variables at the individual level dealt with by previous epidemiological studies, which include lifestyles, preventive awareness and behaviour (including alcohol consumption, smoking and sexual behaviour), communication (including social networks) and consumer activities. Micro-level cultural factors are considered to be under the constant influence of meso-level cultural factors.

The Alameda County Study[11, 12] revealed the relationship between social networks (a micro-level factor) and mortality. It has also been reported that these social networks are related to change of residence or job, or other individual-level (i.e. micro-level) factors, as well as being linked to race, social class, urbanisation and other socio-cultural (i.e. meso-level) factors. Specifically, in the Alameda County Study, it can be construed that the micro-level variables (social networks) affecting the mortality of residents during the follow-up period was affected in turn, by the meso-level factors; that is, the mortality was affected by variables at these two levels. Now, through multilevel analysis, an analytical model unavailable at that time, it has become possible to analyse the effects of interactions between these different levels (cross-level interactions) at the same time.

Association between culture and health

Macro-level culture and health links: comparing cultures

An extremely small number of studies have analysed macro-level cultural variables in the context of physical disease. As mentioned above, from his survey of university students in twenty-one countries worldwide, Bond[10] produced two axes, running between social integration and cultural inwardness, and reputation and social morality. On these, he calculated the average ratings of values for each country. Figure 8.2 is a plotted display of Bond's table[10] prepared by this writer for ease of explanation. Interestingly, there is not a single dot in the second quadrant [cultural inwardness (+), reputation (+)]. The first quadrant [social integration (+), reputation (+)] contains several countries in Europe, and North and South America. The fourth quadrant [social integration (+), social morality (+)] contains a number of Asian countries. On the other hand, the ratings for social integration tend to be higher for so-called developed nations.

Figure 8.2: Positions of selected countries plotted on value dimensions

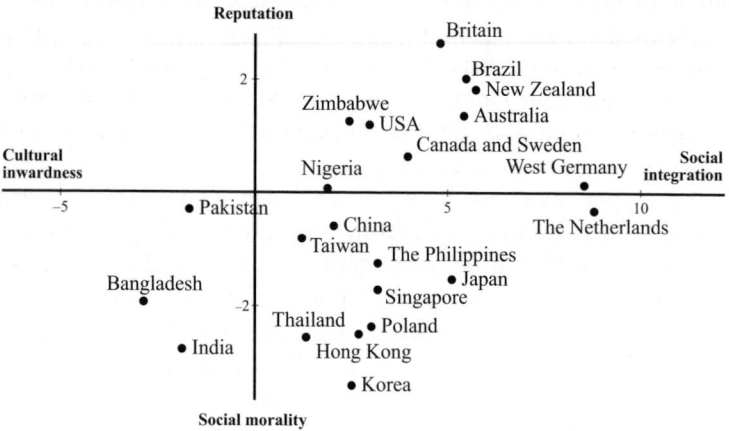

Source: plotted by this author based on Table 2 from Bond (1988)[10].

The appropriateness of this polarisation could be controversial. In fact, Hofstede's bipolarisation (individualism-collectivism)[8], which is often used in cross-cultural comparisons[13] in fields such as social psychology, may be more readily acceptable. However, Bond's work[14] is noteworthy in that using the two dimensions, he further analysed the relationship of the values with disease incidence and gross national product (GNP) for different countries (Table 8.1). There have hardly been any other reports which analyse the potential associations between such macro-level cultural factors and physical health status. In this sense, Bond's work is a valuable reference.

Table 8.1 shows a summary of the reported results. GNP is shown to be associated with demographic indicators, heart disease, colon and breast neoplasm, and arteriosclerosis. After excluding components correlated with GNP, the association between the two-value dimensions and each disease indicator was analysed. Along the social integration-cultural inwardness axis, higher ratings of social integration value are associated with significantly higher incidences of cerebrovascular disease, gastric and duodenal ulcers, and gastric, colon, rectal, sigmoid and anal neoplasm. On the other hand, higher ratings of the cultural inwardness value are not associated with any of the analysed diseases. Along the reputation-social morality axis, higher ratings of the reputation value are associated with significantly higher incidences of acute myocardial infarction and other ischemic heart diseases, as well as colon, rectal, sigmoid and anal neoplasms, and tracheal, bronchial and pulmonary neoplasms. Meanwhile, higher ratings of the social morality value are associated with a significantly higher incidence of hepatic cirrhosis only.

From these results, Bond[14] concludes that, for gastrointestinal ulcers and neoplasms, heart disease and circulatory diseases, cultural areas in which cultural inwardness and social morality are dominant values are healthier than those areas in which social integration and reputation are dominant. On the other hand, neither dimension was associated with longevity, nor with any particular diseases, for example, chronic rheumatic heart disease, atherosclerosis, hypertension, breast cancer or cervical cancer.

Note that these results are based on correlation analysis and multiple regression analysis of countries and have not been proven epidemiologically. However, it is interesting that more diseases have significant associations with these values than with GNP; and that different value dimensions are associated with different diseases. Furthermore, similarities between the diseases associated with GNP and those associated with reputation (after excluding the effects of GNP) suggest a potential association between cultural areas and economic activities.

No report has analysed the potential association between the individualism-collectivism dimension and physical health. However, it could be expected that a 'collectivism' value system[15], which promotes harmony and mutual support among the members of a group, is effective in health promotion and disease prevention[13]. A community-level (i.e. meso-level) analysis of this dimension, when taken together with the results shown in Table 8.1, seems to suggest that 'cultural morality' benefits people's health through a collective process. On the other hand, some have inferred that in a community with poor social support and poor harmony among its members, individuals' coping mechanisms may be upset, resulting in 'cultural isolation' which, in turn, may cause increased cerebrovascular and gastrointestinal diseases[5].

The individualism-collectivism dimension has been used frequently in the fields of psychiatry and psychology. In an individualistic cultural area, the preferred method of psychological treatment is for patients to attempt to delve into themselves with the help of professionals who distance themselves from their patients. Targets of the treatment include a sense of guilt, estrangement or

Table 8.1: Associations between longevity measures, mode of death as a function of Chinese value dimensions and GNP/capita

	Number of countries	Correlation with GNP	Partial correlation controlling for GNP		Variance explained by	
			Social integration	Reputation	GNP	Value dimensions
Longevity measures						
Life expectancy	23	0.76[b]	0.33	−0.32	58[b]	12[a]
Live birth	22	−0.70[b]	−0.40[a]	0.29	49[b]	17[a]
Probability of death before 5	22	−0.74[b]	−0.52[b]	0.26	54[b]	20[b]
Mode of death						
Neoplasm of the rectum, restrosignoid junction and anus	12	0.14	0.72[b]	0.55[a]	2	65[b]
All other malignant neoplasms	12	0.42	0.55[a]	0.43	18	32[a]
Neoplasm of the stomach	12	0.09	0.55[a]	−0.08	1	36[a]
Other circulatory system diseases	12	0.21	0.52[a]	0.07	5	25
Cerebrovascular disease	14	0.61[a]	0.51[a]	0.01	37[a]	19
Ulcer of stomach and duodenum	14	0.39	0.49[a]	0.39	15	9
Neoplasm of the cervix uteri	12	−0.20	0.38	0.20	4	15
Acute myocardial infarction	12	0.56[a]	0.37	0.86[b]	31	53[b]
Other ischemic heart diseases	12	0.74[b]	−0.32	0.84[b]	55[b]	32[a]

	Number of countries	Correlation with GNP	Partial correlation controlling for GNP		Variance explained by	
			Social integration	Reputation	GNP	Value dimensions
Neoplasm of the colon	12	0.77[b]	0.51[a]	0.73[b]	60[b]	26
Neoplasm of the trachea, bronchus and lung	12	0.47	0.32	0.59[b]	22	29
Leukaemia	12	0.08	0.30	0.51	1	29
Cirrhosis of the liver	14	0.37	0.14	−0.50[a]	13	27
Neoplasm of the female breast	12	0.51[a]	0.35	0.49	26	21
Hypertensive disease	14	0.04	0.11	−0.45	0	27
Atherosclerosis	11	−0.62[a]	0.27	−0.17	39[a]	8
Chronic rheumatic heart disease	14	−0.09	0.24	0.05	1	4

Notes. a: $p < 0.05$; b: $p < 0.01$
Source: based on Tables 3 & 4 from Bond (1991)[14].

isolation. In contrast, people in a collective cultural area prefer treatment that is given by professionals who stand close to, and have a personal, emotional relationship with their patients, and who give treatment from a paternalistic, directive, rearer-like position. This treatment focuses more on alleviation of mental agony than on self-understanding[16]. This argument also seems to apply to the treatment of physical diseases. A typical example would be the difference between these two extreme cultural areas in their attitude toward the issue of disclosure to cancer patients of their diagnosis. Another example is health education (including behaviour modification) for AIDS prevention, in which researchers have taken into account the difference between individualistic and collective cultural areas[17].

Meso-level culture and health links: ethnic and migrant communities

In most of the previous studies that analysed meso-level cultural variables, the subjects were immigrants. Specifically, these studies analysed the association between acceptance of the host country's culture and health problems. For example, most of the studies on Asian immigrant populations conducted surveys mainly of immigrants in the USA and their family members and descendants. The surveys were concerned with the levels of adaptation to, and acceptance of, the host country's culture, and analysed the association between these levels and the incidence of health problems. Table 8.2 shows the measures that were used to determine levels of acceptance of the host country's culture by Asian immigrant populations, as tabulated by Talya Salant and Diane Lauderdale in their review[4]. A quick look at these measures shows that the commonly used items describe objective aspects of migration, whereas for other aspects, different cultural variables are used for different objective variables. This suggests that different effects are assessed by different culture-related variables. In addition, a comparison of this table with the three levels of culture (Figure 8.1) reveals that the items listed in the table are of different levels.

Of the seventeen studies which have analysed the association between culture and physical health, only three used scaled measures. These three studies focused on the levels of maintenance of ethnic identity as Korean or Japanese. In most of the unscaled measures used in the remaining fourteen papers, subjects were requested to answer one or two questions on place of birth, period since immigration, Western lifestyles, and so on. In this context,

Table 8.2: Frequency of use of acculturation measures in epidemiological studies on Asian immigrants

	Physical health (n = 17)	Health services use (n = 15)	Mental health/ substance abuse (n = 35)
Multi-item index/scale	3	5	16
Non-scale measures	14	10	19
Items in non-scale measures			
Nativity	6	4	4
Duration of residence/percent of lifetime spent/generation/ age at immigration	6	7	9
Westernisation/western lifestyle (high fat diet, sedentary lifestyle, type A behaviour pattern)	5	0	0
Language (use, proficiency)	1	6	10
Cultural participation (food and media preference, religious activities)	0	0	3
Social relations (support, friends, neighbours)	0	0	5
Other (ethnic identity, material possessions, daily hassles, education, beliefs)	2	3	5

Note: Numbers in parentheses and in the table represent the number of research papers.

Source: Table 1 from Salant & Lauderdale (2003)[4]. Reproduced with permission from Elsevier.

the term 'unscaled' means that, even if the measure contains more than one item, the items are analysed separately and are not taken together as an indicator of the levels of acceptance of the host country's culture.

The process of acceptance of a different culture includes various changes: physical aspects (e.g. housing, streets), biological aspects (e.g. dietary patterns), narrowly-defined cultural aspects (e.g. language, religion) and psychological aspects[18]. However, the previously used items (listed in Table 8.2), such as place of birth and period since immigration, are variables which can be measured more objectively, and they only serve as surrogate variables which are intended to measure, in an extremely indirect manner, certain cultural factors that are assumed to exist and that have changed around these variables. In this sense, it must be said that there is a paucity of research which has sufficiently analysed the effects of acceptance of a different culture on health.

The Japan-Honolulu-San Francisco or Ni-Hon-San Study[19, 20] is a well known epidemiological study on circulatory diseases among Asian immigrant populations, and focused mainly on their acceptance of Western lifestyles (particularly diet). The study analysed how the relevant risk factors and health problems changed in the process of acceptance by Japanese immigrants – whose ethnic ancestors had the lowest incidence of coronary heart disease (CHD) in the world – of the main culture of the host country, the USA, which had the highest occurrence of CHD in the world.

During the period of observation of the Ni-Hon-San Study, the immigrant subjects' dietary patterns changed significantly in that the intake of saturated fat, animal protein and dietary cholesterol increased. As if in concert with these changes, there were increases in the levels of plasma cholesterol, blood glucose, uric acid, body weight and blood pressure. The occurrence of CHD was highest in San Francisco, followed by Honolulu and Japan. On the other hand, with respect to the levels of maintenance of Japanese culture (measured by years of residence in Japan before immigration, frequency of use of Japanese language, and frequency of reading Japanese newspapers), higher levels of maintenance were associated with lower CHD incidence[19, 20].

These results clearly suggest that everyday Japanese customs (meso-level cultural factors) played a suppressive role in the occurrence of CHD as a health problem. In this sense, the study provides a good example of showing the association between culture and health. It is well known that the current upward trend in CHD mortality in Japan has been partly caused by the Westernisation of lifestyles among Japanese people.

Meso- and micro-level culture and health links: religion and lifestyle

As seen in the above examples, it is impossible to analyse meso-level and micro-level cultural factors completely separately because the former factors affect the latter ones. This is particularly true of study methodologies used before multilevel analysis became common. A good example of this is a health survey of Seventh-day Adventists (SDAs).

SDAs have communities all over the world and constitute a unique meso-level culture. A large number of studies have shown that in any country, SDA followers live longer and are healthier than others[21]. According to SDA doctrine, a person's body is considered a temple for the 'Holy Spirit'. For this reason, strict limitations are imposed on the lifestyle of SDA followers. Their main diet includes unrefined foods, grains, vegetable protein, fruit and vegetables. They are supposed to refrain from consuming alcohol, tobacco and other luxuries. In other words, the meso-level cultural factor of 'being an SDA' is itself a direct determinant of micro-level factors (e.g. aspects of personal lifestyle).

It has also been shown that SDA communities have lower cancer rates and that there is a 'dose-response' relationship between the levels of compliance with an SDA lifestyle and health risks. These findings show the significance of micro-level cultural factors (personal lifestyles) for health, as well as the difficulty of analysing them completely separately from the effects of a meso-level cultural factor (religious beliefs). Cultural factors (of a higher level) which have been internalised are observed through lifestyles, and this is another characteristic of higher-level cultural factors.

Micro-level culture and health links: youth lifestyles

I have thus far focused on the association between lifestyle-related diseases and culture. Below, cultural factors are discussed in the context of infectious diseases. Amid the downward trend in the number of new HIV carriers in most developed countries, Japan is one of the few with an increasing number of new HIV carriers[22]. When we think of this increase, the highest risk group is youth (particularly females). Youth culture (a micro-level factor) is a typical example of a culture unique to a specific generation. It is a culture constructed by youth (from puberty to adolescence) based on their own values, which are often different from existing values. Sexual behaviour represents an individual's lifestyle but is also greatly affected by 'sexual culture'[23, 24]. This sexual culture constitutes part of youth culture.

In present day Japan, information on sexual behaviour is distributed through various media. Compared to only two decades ago, the development of mobile phones and the Internet has made it easier for young people to directly obtain information and distribute it to others. This development of technology has brought significant changes in youth culture. Specifically, in former times, there was a variety of information that was accessible only to so-called 'underground' groups. Nowadays, such information can be distributed worldwide in an instant. Whether you live in a city or elsewhere, you can now receive and respond to all kinds of information.

Arguably, this situation has had greatest impact on information about sex. In the process of their socialisation, young people can easily construct information networks. This allows them to be exposed to an enormous amount of sexual information and to construct easy sexual networks before they have established their own identities. Because of their exposure to abundant information inappropriate for their age, an increasing number of young people have developed inappropriate behaviour where they act before they think, instead of acting after sensible consideration of a situation.

It seems that this sexual culture has been defining sexual lifestyles (a micro-level cultural factor), has been changing the understanding of gender roles in marriage, childbirth and childrearing (a meso-level cultural factor), and furthermore, has been changing the social norm-value system (a macro-level factor). Certainly, these changes have occurred partly due to the influence of Western culture. Similarly to the aforementioned acceptance of a different culture, the dynamism of a culture usually means that a change first occurs in low-level cultural factors and then spreads to upper-level cultural factors. Once a new sexual culture has been formed and spread to the upper levels, it is extremely difficult to restore the former, orderly culture. This is why barriers to the prevention of sexually transmitted diseases are high. In any case, the association between culture and infectious diseases is very easy to understand because culture characteristically promotes a certain value system or behaviour pattern.

Globalisation and social epidemiology

Amid the worldwide trend of globalisation and in the wake of the explosive spread of socioeconomic activities and information technology, our culture has been facing pressure at various levels. As described in the previous section, resulting changes start from micro-level cultural factors. In other words, they first occur in the most minute aspects of lifestyle. This suggests, as described in the section on ethnic and migrant communities, the possibility that these changes may affect the development of lifestyle-related diseases and other health problems in a relatively short time.

Globalisation, through multinational companies, for instance, will result in a work culture whose upper-level cultural factors are different from those of a local company. 'Uncertainty avoidance' (including perfectionism), which is a macro-level cultural factor, ethnicity, which is a meso-level factor, and workplace ethics, corporate culture and other micro-level factors will often coexist in the same workplace. This will naturally result in situations where the subculture may be accepted or denied by the main culture, or where a foreign culture must be accepted. These situations will affect employees' health through psychosocial stress.

These changes that will be brought about by globalisation may have effects on various aspects of people's everyday lives. There is a paucity of information for us to guess the degree to which these effects may influence macro-level cultural factors. However, the collective values in Japan, for example, have already become weaker than before, and this trend is expected to continue in the future.

Although I refrained from mentioning it in this chapter for want of space, mental disorders (including drug abuse), mental/psychological health status, prejudice and health-care seeking behaviour seem to be affected greatly by upper-level cultural factors (e.g. spirituality). Globalisation allows us to collect information from all over the world. Making good use of this phenomenon may enable us to simultaneously analyse the effects of macro-, meso- and micro-level cultural factors on various health-care issues dealt with by social epidemiology. On the other hand, to make effective interventions (i.e. take health care measures) based on findings thus far obtained, we should start with changing specific behaviour patterns at the micro-level (i.e. individual behavioural factors) and proceed to higher levels in a step-by-step manner.

Literature

1 Tylor, E. B. (1871), *Primitive culture: researches into the development of mythology, philosophy, religion, language, art and custom*, London: John Murray & Co. [Republished in 1974, New York: Gordon Press]
2 Kroeber, A. L. and C. Kluckhohn (1952), *Culture: a critical review of concepts and definitions*, Cambridge (Massachusetts): Peabody Museum.
3 UNESCO (2002), UNESCO Universal Declaration on Cultural Diversity.
4 Salant, T. and D. S. Lauderdale (2003), 'Measuring culture: a critical review of acculturation and health in Asian immigrant populations', *Social Science and Medicine*, 57, pp. 71–90.
5 MacLachlan, M. (1997), *Culture and health: Chichester*, England: John Wiley & Sons Ltd.
6 Ahdieh, L. and R. A. Hahn (1996), 'Use of terms "race", "ethnicity" and "national origin": a review of articles in the American Journal of Public Health, 1980–89', *Ethnicity and Health*, 1, pp. 95–98.

7 Schoendorf, K. C., C. J. R. Hogue, J. C. Kleinman and D. L. Rowley (1992), 'Mortality among infants of black as compared with white college-educated parents', *New England Journal of Medicine*, 326, pp. 1522–1526.
8 Hofstede, G. (1980), *Culture's consequences: international differences in work-related values*, Beverly Hills: Sage.
9 Hofstede, G. (1991), *Cultures and organizations*, London: Harper-Collins Publishers.
10 Bond, M. H. (1988), 'Finding universal dimensions of individual variation in multicultural studies of values: the Rokeach and Chinese values survey', *Journal of Personality and Social Psychology*, 55, pp. 1009–1015.
11 Berkman, L. F. and L. Breslow (1979), 'Social networks, host resistance, and mortality: a nine-year follow-up study of Alameda County residents', *American Journal of Epidemiology*, 109, pp. 186–204.
12 Berkman, L. F. and L. Breslow (1983), *Health and ways of living: the Alameda County Study*, New York: Oxford University Press.
13 Triandis, H. C., R. Bontempo, M. J. Villareal, M. Asai and N. Lucca (1988), 'Individualism and collectivism: cross-cultural perspectives on self in-group relationships', *Journal of Personality and Social Psychology*, 54, pp. 323–338.
14 Bond, M. H. (1991), 'Chinese values and health: a cultural-level examination', *Psychology and Health*, 5, pp. 137–152.
15 Hofstede, G. (1986), 'Cultural differences in teaching and learning', *International Journal of Intercultural Relations*, 10, pp. 301–320.
16 Draguns, J. G. (1990), 'Applications of cross-cultural psychology in the field of mental health', in R. W. Brislin (ed), *Applied Cross-Cultural Psychology*, Newbury Park: Sage, pp. 302–324.
17 Midha, A. (1998), 'The need to redefine the practice of health promotion in the United Kingdom', *Health Policy*, 44, pp. 19–30.
18 Ilola, L. M. (1990), 'Culture and health', in R. W. Brislin (ed), *Applied Cross-Cultural Psychology*, Newbury Park: Sage, pp. 278–301.
19 Kato, H., J. Tillotson, M. Z. Nichaman, G. G. Rhoads and H. B. Hamilton (1973), 'Epidemiologic studies of coronary heart disease and stroke in Japanese men living in Japan, Hawaii and California', *American Journal of Epidemiology*, 97, pp. 372–384.
20 Kagan, A., B. R. Harris, W. Winkelstein Jr., K. G. Johnson, H. Kato, S. L. Syme, G. G. Rhoads, M. L. Gay, M. Z. Nichaman, H. B. Hamilton and J. Tillotson (1974), 'Epidemiologic studies of coronary heart disease and stroke in Japanese men living Japan, Hawaii and California: demographic, physical, dietary and biochemical characteristics', *Journal of Chronic Disease*, 27, pp. 345–364.
21 Fraser, G. E., W. L. Beeson and R. L. Phillips (1991), 'Diet and lung cancer in California Seventh-day Adventists', *American Journal of Epidemiology*, 133, pp. 683–693.
22 The Committee on AIDS Trends, Ministry of Health, Labour and Welfare of Japan (2005), *Heisei 16-nen eizu hassei dōkō nenpō; Kōsei Rōdōshō Eizu Dōkō Iinkai hōkoku* (The 2004 report on AIDS trends; a report by the Committee on AIDS Trends, Ministry of Health, Labour and Welfare of Japan), Ministry of Health, Labour and Welfare of Japan.

23 Marston, C. (2004), 'Gendered communication among young people in Mexico: implications for sexual health interventions', *Social Science and Medicine*, 59, pp. 445–456.
24 Shoveller, J. A., J. L. Johnson, D. B. Langille and T. Mitchell (2004), 'Socio-cultural influences on young people's sexual development', *Social Science and Medicine*, 59, pp. 473–487.

9 Social Relationships and Health

Katsunori Kondō

Introduction

In this chapter, the links between health and social relationships (including social networks, social support and social capital) are discussed. Factors that influence health can be presented at several levels. Figure 9.1[1] shows the determinants of health, with the micro-level factors placed on the inside and the macro-level factors on the outside. The biomedical model, which focuses on the innermost level, the 'individual as a life form', attempts to explain health according to factors within the individual. In contrast, social epidemiology focuses on the effects at the second level, 'personal socioeconomic factors', and the third level, 'society as the environment'.

Social relationships influencing health can be viewed at two levels at least. One is the second level in Figure 9.1, which is the 'individual level'; but the most notable relationships are personal human relationships. Social relationships on this level include: marriage, the type of family living arrangements, relatives, friends and other forms of social networks and social support.

The other is the third level in Figure 9.1, which is the 'society (as the environment) level'. For instance, a serious economic recession could lead to an increase in depression sufferers and suicide victims among people who lose their jobs due to increased unemployment and business failures. Similarly, living in a community with a high crime rate could increase exposure to physical risks and anxiety, which could in turn, result in poorer psychological health. Thus, a person can be influenced by their social environment at the 'society level' beyond the 'individual level'.

In this chapter, I discuss social relationships at the 'individual level' in the following 3 sections, and social relationships at the 'society level', for example, as social capital, in the final section. In each section, I outline various concepts involved, summarise the results of previous studies with some mention of our own data, and discuss our hypotheses for why these social relationships influence

Figure 9.1: Hierarchical structure of the determinants of health

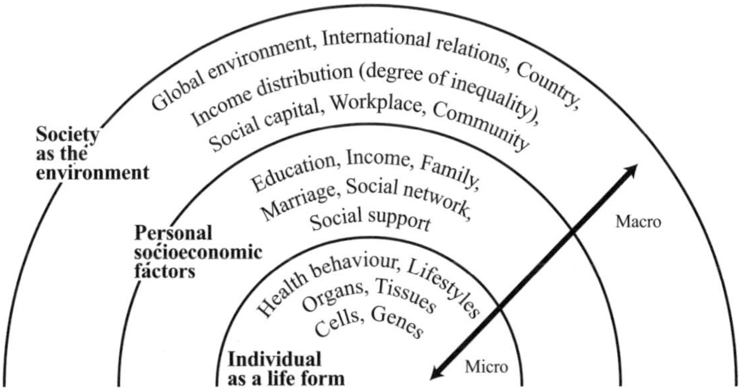

```
                Global environment, International relations, Country,
                    Income distribution (degree of inequality),
                      Social capital, Workplace, Community
  Society
  as the                 Education, Income, Family,
  environment             Marriage, Social network,
                              Social support                         Macro
           Personal
           socioeconomic
           factors      Health behaviour, Lifestyles
                          Organs, Tissues
                            Cells, Genes
                     Individual
                     as a life form        Micro
```

Source: Kondō (2005 p.150)[1]. Revised.

health, as well as criticisms to be addressed and research topics to be dealt with in the future.

Concepts involved in individual-level social relationships

Recent years have seen a remarkable increase in the number of scientific papers on personal relationships and health. For instance, searching the Medline database using the keyword 'social support' produces only three hits for 1980. The number of hits increases to 777 for 1990 and then to as many as 1,421 for 2000. One reason for the increase is the fact that this topic readily attracts interdisciplinary attention. If you focus on the relationship between social support and mortality, there are research topics in epidemiology and public hygiene. If you focus on social support's connections with smoking, exercise habits and other health behaviour, there are research topics in health sciences (health sociology) and behavioural science. Various links have been made in other disciplines as well, including occupational health, psychiatry, psychology, sociology and gerontology.

Previous studies have found that compared to those who have rich social networks, those who are socially isolated, or specifically, those who are unmarried, who have poor relationships with their family members, relatives and friends and who do not participate in group activities, are likely to be in poorer health, both physically and psychologically[5,6].

Since the focus is different in different disciplines, there is no perfect consensus on the relevant definitions, concepts involved or measuring methods in the area of social support[2-4]. Table 9.1 shows a summary of concepts and classifications on which a reasonable consensus has been reached.

Family: spouses and household types

Family members, particularly a spouse, are usually the people who are closest to you. However, it is inadequate to simply focus on whether or not people have a spouse, and divide them into married and single. Single people may be unmarried, divorced or widowed. Married people may be in their first or second marriage. As described below, it has been found that these marital statuses have different associations with health. In addition, it has been revealed that among married people, poor satisfaction with conjugal relations is associated with depression.

Furthermore, the potential influence of household type should be taken into account. For example, it may make a difference whether an elderly person who has recently lost his/her spouse lives alone or with his/her child's family.

Social networks

'Social network' is a concept for quantitatively evaluating the structural aspects of personal relationships. Items for evaluation include how often a person sees or communicates by telephone or mail with people in several categories (e.g. family members who live together, relatives, friends, community members, religious community members and volunteer group members). This social network is the provider of social support discussed in the following subsection. Social networks and social support are sometimes referred to as 'social support-networks'[3] or 'social ties'[4].

Social support

An evaluation that focuses on the functional, qualitative aspects of someone's personal relationships is often referred to as 'social support', as distinct from a 'social network'. Social support has subordinate concepts as listed in Table 9.1. First, by focusing on its contents, social support can be divided into emotional support,

Table 9.1: Social network and social support

Social network
Evaluation of structure and quantity of networks with others
Being a provider of social support
Social support
Evaluation of functions and quality of support to others
Contents of support
Emotional support
Instrumental support
Informational support
Types of support
Objective support
Existing support
Support in use
Subjective support
Known or expected support
If focusing on the appropriateness of support
Positive support
Negative support
If focusing on exchange of support
Receipt of support
Provision of support

Source: Kondō (2005)[1].

instrumental support (e.g. nursing care and financial support) and informational support. It can also be divided into support which is actually in use and support which is not currently in use but known to be available if needed. In addition, social support may not always be received positively or seen as desirable by the user. It could be support which is uninvited by the receiver and viewed negatively. Related to this idea is the suggestion that a person is likely to feel a stronger sense of efficacy when providing support than when receiving it[4].

Below I review the relationship between marriage and household type, on the one hand, and health, on the other, followed by some discussion of social support-networks.

Marriage and health

The family sociologist Catherine E. Ross and her colleagues have made a comprehensive literature review of the impact of the family on health, from four aspects: marriage, childrearing, women's employment and the family's socioeconomic status[7]. Below I outline their review findings on the relationship between marriage and health.

According to the review, married people are physically healthier, have a greater psychological well-being, and have lower mortality than unmarried, divorced, separated or widowed people (hereinafter referred to as 'single people'). These benefits of marriage are seen in both men and women, but more prominently in men.

Health of single people

The mortality of single people compared to married people is higher by 50% in women and by as much as 150% in men. The prominent causes of death include lung cancer and hepatic cirrhosis (which are likely to be affected by a person's smoking and alcohol consumption status, respectively), suicide and unexpected accidents. A selection bias could have existed in that the unhealthier a person (or his/her behaviour) is, the less likely he/she is to be married. However, this cannot explain all the differences[7, 8].

Ross's findings are based on data obtained overseas, where most single people live alone. Does this apply to Japan, where it is not uncommon for single people to live with their parents until they marry? Are single people in Japan more likely than their married counterparts to suffer from loneliness, anxiety or depression?

We analysed the relationship between marital status and psychological health among 1,196 Japanese women aged between 29 and 39[9]. We calculated the odds ratios of reporting any mental problem, such as depression, experienced during the previous year. When the odds ratio for women in their first marriage is set at 1, the odds ratios for unmarried women, divorced women and remarried women were 4.9, 8.1 and 10.2, respectively. These results confirmed that among Japanese women aged between 29 and 39, unmarried, divorced or remarried women are also approximately five to ten times more likely to have mental problems than women in their first marriage. There have been other reports from Japan showing that remarried people are more likely than divorced people to be in poor mental health, but this tendency cannot be seen in the USA[9]. This is a prospective future topic for international comparative research.

Influence of a spouse's death

It has been found that one may experience depression and/or anxiety as a normal response to the death of a spouse. Not only that, the death of a spouse is associated with increased mortality of the surviving spouse. According to one report, this increase peaks immediately (within six months) after the spouse's death, and depending on the cause of death, the mortality of the surviving spouse increases 5–150%[7].

Satisfaction with marriage/conjugal relations and health

Hence, is marriage always good for a couple's health? Even if all married people appear the same in that they have a spouse, the spouse's function, so to say, is varied, as seen in the expression 'separate lives under the same roof'. Let me outline our Aichi Gerontological Evaluation Study (AGES) project[10], in which we attempted to analyse this point using the criterion of 'marital satisfaction'[11].

The subjects were a representative general sample of elderly people (aged 65 and over) in fifteen municipalities. We excluded people who had been certified by municipal governments as being eligible for receiving care under long term care insurance. The sample size was 32,891 subjects (collection rate: 55.2%). Marital satisfaction was checked on a six-level scale and ranked on a three-level scale (high, medium or low).

Married people accounted for 89.0% and 56.1% of a total of 13,295 men and a total of 15,634 women, respectively. Widowed or divorced subjects represented 10.4% and 41.7% of men and women, respectively, with the remaining ones being unmarried. Of the married subjects, a greater proportion of men (67.1%) than women (52.2%) showed a high level of marital satisfaction.

We assessed depression in the subjects using the 15-item Geriatric Depression Scale (GDS), whose validity and reliability had been checked (depression was defined as ≥ 10 points). The proportion

Figure 9.2: Marital status, marital satisfaction and depression (≥ 10 points in GDS; results based on a general linear model adjusted for age)

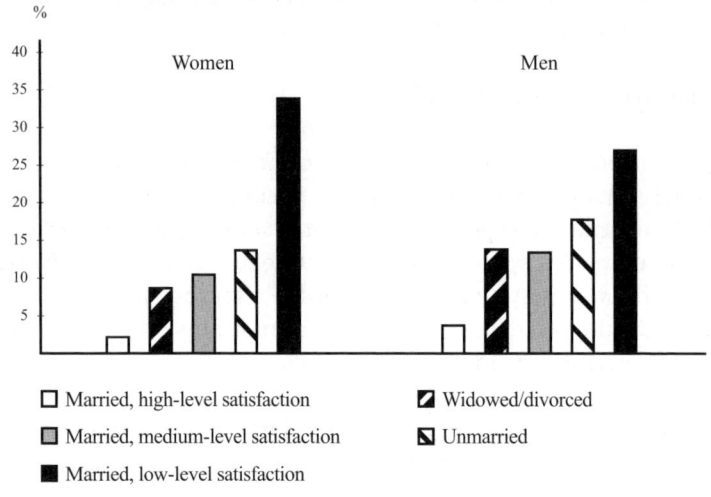

Source: modified from Suemori (2007)[11].

of subjects with depression tended to be higher in the following order: 1) unmarried, 2) widowed/divorced, and 3) married. However, interesting results were obtained when we divided the married people into three groups according to the level of marital satisfaction (Figure 9.2). The high-level satisfaction group had extremely low incidences of depression (3.8% and 2.3% of men and women, respectively). In contrast, the low-level satisfaction group had higher incidences of depression (27.0% and 33.6% of men and women) than the widowed/divorced group or the unmarried group. In the medium-level satisfaction group, the proportion of men with depression was slightly lower than men in the widowed/divorced group, whereas in women the corresponding proportion was higher than the widowed/divorced group. There is a Japanese saying: 'Widowed women become healthier'. The above figures support this opinion within the low- and medium-level marital satisfaction groups.

Concerning the association between household structure and depression, 17.7% of men living alone had depression, a proportion significantly higher than in the other groups (5.5% and 9.6%). For women, the corresponding proportion was 9.1%, which was not as high as for men, but still somewhat higher than the other groups.

Why does marriage mean good health?

Attempts have been made to explain this phenomenon from two aspects[7]: 1) social support (mainly emotional support), and 2) economic stability.

Social support
Previous research has proposed four mechanisms by which spousal social support brings health benefits[7].

The first is emotional support. This brings benefits through the perception that your spouse is concerned about you, loves you and regards you as a valuable person. Married people are more likely than single people to answer that they receive social support, including this emotional support. Emotional support has also been known to keep down incidences of depression, anxiety, certain diseases and mortality.

The second mechanism is through healthy lifestyles. Married people are more likely to quit smoking, be on a well-balanced diet, and avoid alcohol abuse.

Thirdly, married people are more likely than single people to seek medical advice early and to receive treatment early.

Fourthly, social support promotes recovery from illness. It has been found that having a family promotes recovery from emotional disturbance, such as depression following myocardial infarction or breast cancer.

Economic stability
The second pathway of action is economic stability. Data on household incomes show that married households tend to have a higher income per person than unmarried households. As described in Chapter 2, being economically wealthy has positive effects on health.

Social support-networks

'The evidence that social support is beneficial to health and that social isolation leads to ill health is now considerable.'[5]

Social networks

Between 1965 and 1974, a large-scale cohort study was conducted with 4,775 subjects aged between 30 and 69 living in Alameda

County, California[12]. At the start of follow-up, the subjects were questioned whether they had four social ties: marriage, contact with relatives and friends, church activities, and other formal or informal group activities. Based on responses to the questions, a social network index was calculated. After nine years, results showed that the mortality of people with low index scores, which indicate social isolation, was 1.9 to 3 times higher than those with high scores. As people who are prone to illness or in low social classes may be more likely to be socially isolated, the results were statistically adjusted for potential confounders, including physical health, socioeconomic status, race, smoking, alcohol consumption, physical exercise, obesity, life satisfaction and use of preventive health care. After adjusting for all of these, social isolation was still found to be a predictor of earlier death.

Subsequently, a large number of cohort studies have been conducted to corroborate the relationship between social networks and death (Figure 9.3). Similar results[4-6] have been reported not only from America[6, 13-15] but also from Japan[16, 17], Finland, Sweden and Britain[18].

Social support

On the other hand, a close look at the studies on social support reveals that they have produced inconsistent results. There are at least two conceivable reasons for this. First, people who receive support include those who already have a weakness of some kind which makes them require support. There is a possibility that their poor prognosis may produce unexpected results that appear to show an association between support and poor prognosis. In order to clarify this point, we need to accumulate analyses which exclude those who have any weakness from the subjects of a cohort study. Another reason is the potential significance of the balance between the two aspects of support, 'receiving' and 'providing'.

Thus, we studied these possibilities using data from the AGES project[19, 20].

First, we analysed the degree to which elderly people receive and/or provide emotional and instrumental support. Depending on the subjects' answers to the following questions, we divided them into four groups: a) those who both receive and provide social support; b) those who only receive social support; c) those who only provide social support; and d) those who neither receive nor provide social support. The questions on emotional support were: 'Do you have

Figure 9.3: Social networks and mortality

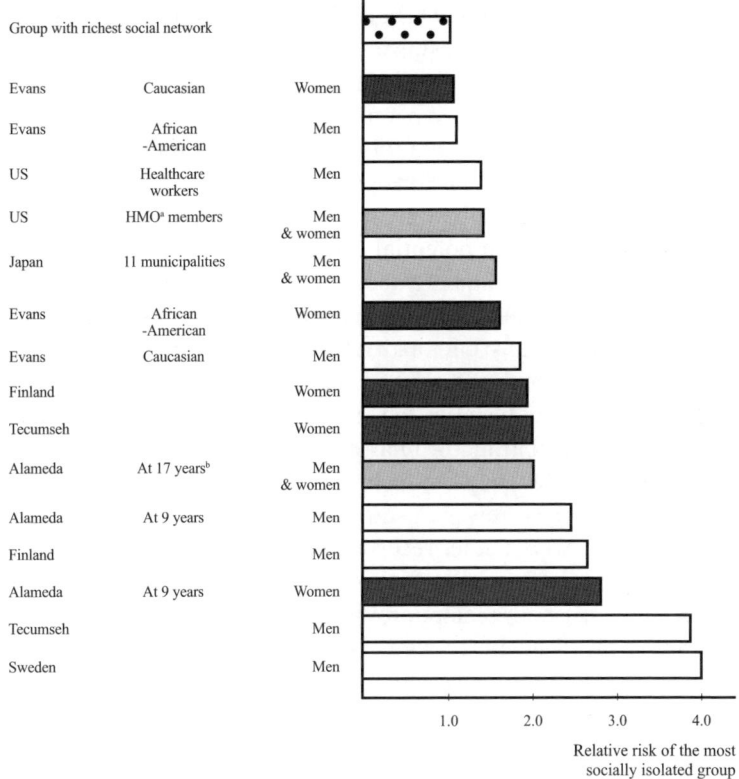

Note: Based on data presented by House in graphic form, with the addition of data from four articles published subsequently. Names other than country names are US county names. Graphic data show relative risk when the mortality of the group with the richest social network is set at 1.

a: HMO (Health Maintenance Organization).

b: Values for subjects aged 38–49.

Source: Kondō (2005 p.60)[1].

anyone who is willing to listen to your worries and complaints ...?' (i.e. receipt of support) and 'Do you have anyone whose worries and complaints ... you are willing to listen to?' (i.e. provision of support). The questions on instrumental support were: 'Do you have anyone who would nurse or take care of you ... if you were sick in bed for a few days?' (i.e. receipt of support) and 'Do you have anyone whom you would nurse or take care of ... if he/she were sick in bed for a few days? (i.e. provision of support).

The proportion of subjects who both received and provided support was highest. Of all subjects, 79.3% both received and provided emotional support, and 88.8% received and provided instrumental support. These were followed by Group (b), those who only receive support (emotional, 11.0%; instrumental, 5.2%); and Group (c) those who only provide support (emotional, 4.0%; instrumental, 3.3%). Those who neither receive nor provide support, Group (d), were few in number (emotional, 5.7%; instrumental, 2.7%).

Next, we studied the potential associations between these four patterns of receipt and/or provision of social support, on the one hand, and depression (≥ 10 points in the 15-item GDS) and self-rated health in elderly people, on the other. The results showed that subjects who both receive and provide support, Group (a), had the best mental health status. For instance, regarding instrumental support, the age-adjusted proportions of subjects with depression were 6.3% of those who both receive and provide suppport, 15.0% of those who only receive, 22.4% of those who only provide, and 28.0% of those who neither receive nor provide ($p < 0.001$).

However, a cross-sectional study does not allow researchers to find out whether poor receipt/provision of social support results in psychological ill health or conversely, if psychological ill health results in poor receipt/provision of social support. Thus, we followed the subjects for two years and analysed data. From the results, we have confirmed that poor provision of social support precedes ill health and is associated with a tendency towards health disadvantages[20].

These results show that for the good health of the elderly, it is more desirable for them to both provide and receive support than to only provide or only receive support, much less doing neither, in their personal relationships.

Furthermore, social support among the elderly was also associated with age and socioeconomic status. Younger age, longer years of education, and higher income tended to be associated with more social support. The effects of these many confounders need to be examined in future analyses.

How do social support-networks influence health?

The effects of social support-networks on health have been analysed from two perspectives: the main (or direct) effect and the stress-relieving (or indirect) effect[3, 4, 6]. The main effect represents a concept that, regardless of whether or not a person is under stress, a social support-network acts mainly to improve his/her health; and conversely, lack of a social support-network (social isolation) acts as a stressor itself, and has negative effects on health. Alternatively, the stress-relieving effect represents a concept that if one is exposed to a stressor, social support acts mainly to buffer its effects. Previous studies have shown that social support has both of these effects.

Future research challenges

A number of research challenges have been outlined[4, 6], but let me mention only four of them.

The first challenge is to organise various similar concepts (Table 9.1) based on theoretical and empirical studies. The social support-network idea has various aspects, but we need to organise previous findings to find out whether it is necessary to analyse all the aspects, and then which aspects are more important. In addition, recent studies seem to show that if a comparison is made between analyses from a structural point of view and those from a functional view, the latter generally seem to have produced more consistent results. If a structural factor (e.g. being married) can be described from a functional aspect (e.g. marital satisfaction), it may be better able to explain the phenomenon in question.

The second challenge is to make measuring methods more sophisticated. In our attempts to overcome the first challenge, we have to ask more and detailed questions to collect detailed information. However, this results in increased non-response rates. We need to improve our methods of measurement and analysis. For example, we need to formulate questions that produce consistent results, and that are sensitive and easy to answer, as well as needing to improve methods of processing variables.

The third challenge is to elucidate the pathways through which individuals' social relationships influence their health. Even if there is an association between social relationships and health, and cohort studies have proved a temporal anterior-posterior relationship between them, this will not necessarily mean that there is a direct causal relationship between them. In addition, we need to study effective intervention approaches. For these reasons, it is necessary to clarify how social relationships influence health.

The fourth challenge is to develop intervention approaches and examine their effects. Even if individuals' social relationships have a causal association with their health, and even if the pathways through which social relationships influence health are clarified, this will not necessarily mean social relationships can be manipulated to improve health levels. There are several issues to be addressed, such as what interventions can be made, if they are practical, and how much they can be manipulated.

Society as environment: social capital

Apart from the 'individual-level' social relationships described thus far, there are also 'society-level' social relationships. These can also be labelled 'society as environment'. There are several aspects to 'society as environment' that are currently attracting attention in social epidemiology. Examples include: the 'relative income hypothesis' (see Chapter 3), that is, that significant income inequality in a society is associated with low health levels of people living in the society; also the influence on health of health care access (see Chapter 4); and social capital. Of these, this section focuses on social capital.

Concepts related to social capital

As shown in Table 9.2, there are various definitions of social capital[21, 22]. For instance, the World Bank says 'Social capital refers to the institutions, relationships, and norms that shape the quality and quantity of a society's social interactions... Social capital is not just the sum of the institutions which underpin a society – it is the glue that holds them together.' Putnam[23] defines it as characteristics at the 'society level', that is, 'features of social organization, such as trust, norms, and networks that can improve the efficiency of society by facilitating coordinated actions.' Putnam describes social capital as solidarity by which people help each other to overcome a problem by bringing wisdom, materials, funds and labour together. Putnam further notes that this kind of experience produces social capital of a higher level and strengthens cooperation among people.

On the other hand, some of the definitions of social capital made in such disciplines as sociology (Coleman) and business administration (Baker) include the social network idea[24]. In social epidemiology and public health, more researchers use the term 'social capital' to refer to social networks and social support at the social/organisational level as compared to those at the individual level[22, 25–28].

Table 9.2: Definitions of social capital appearing in research

	Year	Outline
Lydia Judson Hanifan, American educator	1916	Social capital is defined as goodwill, fellowship, mutual sympathy, and social intercourse. Hanifan uses this concept to explain the importance of a school's involvement in the community.
Pierre Bourdieu, French sociologist	1986	Social capital is defined as an individual's network, etc. to access power and resources. An individual's social capital is viewed as a determinant of his/her education or employment opportunities. Bourdieu uses the concept of social capital from the viewpoint that it is a mechanism to divide people into, and entrench, social classes.
James S. Coleman, American sociologist	1988 1990	Social capital is defined as social structure and systems to cause individuals to take coordinated action. Coleman explains the mechanism by which reasonable persons take coordinated action using the concepts of trust, norms of reciprocity, and social network.
Robert D. Putnam, American political scientist	1993	Using the concept of social network, Putnam explains the difference in system performance between local governments in northern Italy and those in southern Italy. Putnam defines social capital as characteristics of a social system, such as 'trust', 'norms' and 'network', and notes that social capital increases the efficiency of society by promoting people's coordinated action.

Source: Kondō (2005 p.139)[1].

There are a number of concepts similar to social capital. Examples include 'the culture and capabilities of your organization'[24]; collective efficacy[29]; community solution[30]; and social integration/cohesion[26]. In this chapter, I limit my discussion to the community level but use the term 'social capital' in a somewhat broader sense that includes the community's ability to unify its members and to solve problems.

Social capital and its growing popularity

Over the last decade, social capital has attracted more and more attention[25, 28] in some areas of public health, including health promotion[31]. This trend was triggered by reports that a richer social capital among residents in a community is associated with better subjective health[32, 33] and lower mortality[34, 35].

This concept of social capital originated[26, 37] in sociology[36] and politics[23, 26]. There have also been reports that a richer social capital in a community is associated with better school performances among children, reduced TV viewing by children and a lower school dropout rate[36]; and generally, a lower crime rate[36, 38, 39], a better performance by local government, and higher numbers of childcare facilities and general practitioners for the population size[23]. Richer social capital has also been associated with higher organisational productivity and higher economic growth rates in the fields of business administration[24], social development[21, 40] and economics[41]. In a sense, social capital has become a vogue expression in a variety of disciplines.

Social capital and health indicators

A study from the USA shows an association between social capital and health. In Figure 9.4[34], the horizontal axis represents an indicator of mutual trust, which is an indicator of social capital. The vertical axis represents age-adjusted mortality. The figure shows that the closer to the left a community is plotted, the richer its social capital (i.e. the smaller the proportion of people who do not trust others), and the lower its mortality.

In Canada, this association between richer social capital and higher health levels has also been reported in studies on mortality rates[35] and self-rated health[32] (which is known to be a predictor of death). According to Kimberly Lochner and colleagues[42], studies on the relationships between social capital and suicide can be traced as far back as a report by David Durkheim in the 19th century, which showed that the higher the social integration of a community, the lower the number of suicide cases experienced by the community. In addition, in the USA an association has been reported between a richer social capital in a community and a lower number of deaths by homicide[38, 39].

There is another reason for the attention paid to social capital in the context of health. An association has been found between social capital and degrees of income disparity. Previous reports have shown associations between severe income inequality (i.e. wider income disparity) on the one hand, and high mutual distrust, low mutual support and a poor sense of solidarity on the other[34, 36, 38]. In other words, severer income inequality is associated with poorer social capital. It has been pointed out that it may be the mechanism of the

Figure 9.4: Age-adjusted mortality and lack of interpersonal trust

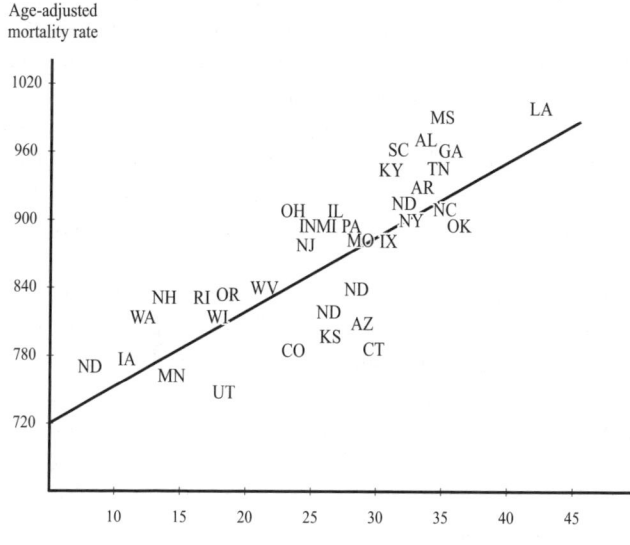

Note: Capital letters represent the abbreviations of US states.
Source: Kawachi, et al (1997)[34].

'relative income hypothesis' (see Chapter 3) that means the severer the income disparities in a community or country, the lower the health levels of the residents[22, 25].

Social capital and elderly abuse

It is very interesting that social capital is associated with so many phenomena. We also analysed the relationships between social capital of a community and elderly abuse, using data from the AGES project[43]. Since previous studies had shown an association between social capital and crimes, we assumed that social capital may be associated with abuse of the elderly as well.

The subjects were a representative sample of the general elderly population who were 65 years old and over, and had not been certified as in need of long term care (collection rate, 50.2%; n = 17,269), and all elderly persons who required long term care and were using home care services (collection rate, 81.4%; n = 5920) in five municipalities for which school district data were available. Each municipality was divided into four to six districts based on the primary school or junior high school districts, so that all districts had a similar sample size. For a total of 24 districts, the following values were calculated.

The variables of social capital were obtained from the general elderly population survey and comprised 'general trust', 'norms of reciprocity' and 'number of networks (organisations and associations) the subject participated in'. Specifically, the variables were formulated from answers to the following questions, in each case based on previous studies. For general trust, the subjects were requested to answer 'Yes' or 'No' or 'Depends' to the question, 'Do you generally think people are reliable?'. For norms of reciprocity, they were asked to answer 'Yes' or 'No' or 'Depends' to the question, 'Do you think people usually try to help others?'. For each variable, the percentage of subjects who answered 'No' to the question was calculated. Regarding participation in networks, the subjects were requested to mention the volunteer groups, clubs for the elderly, hobby clubs, etc. in which they participated. The average number of groups or clubs per person was calculated.

At the same time, the proportion of 'inappropriate care' was calculated based on assessments provided by care managers who were in charge of elderly in need of long term care. 'Inappropriate care' included abuse in a narrow sense and also neglect. In the assessment of abuse in a narrow sense, cases with, or with an undeniable possibility of psychological and/or economic abuse, were entered into the 'abuse group'. Regarding neglect, care managers were requested to assess the quality of care giving from four aspects: 'personal care', 'certain basic movements', 'daily household chores' and 'weekly household chores'. Cases which were assessed as 'problematic' or 'possible' were entered into the 'problematic group'. Cases in the 'abuse group' and/or the 'problematic group' were then put into the 'inappropriate care group'[44].

The results showed that for all three indicators of social capital, poorer social capital was associated with a larger number of subjects in the inappropriate care group. Figure 9.5 shows one example. School districts with a larger number of subjects who answered 'People are not reliable' had a larger number of subjects in the inappropriate care group ($r = 0.56$, $p < 0.01$). A similar correlation was found for norms of reciprocity ($r = 0.49$, $p < 0.05$) and participation in networks ($r = 0.43$, $p < 0.05$).

This association would be expected if 'inappropriate care' and social capital were assessed by the same person, due to the likelihood that persons who have witnessed abuse would answer 'People are

Figure 9.5: Social capital and 'inappropriate care' (by school districts)

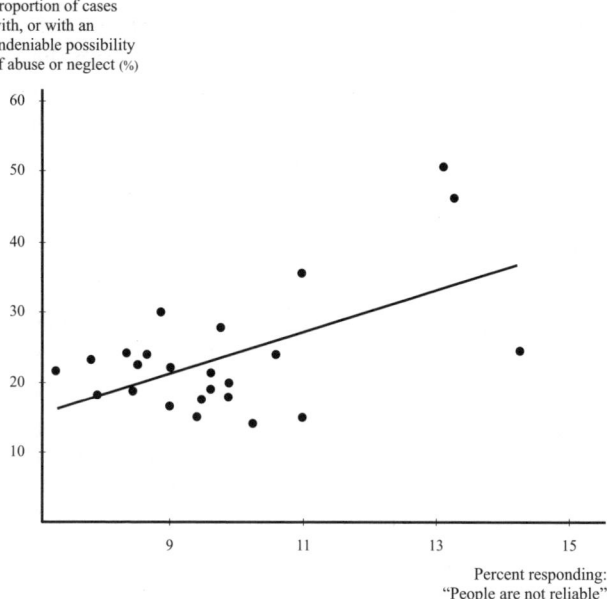

not reliable'. However, this analysis is characterised by the complete independence of the assessors of one variable from those of the other. It is interesting that despite this independence, an association was found between the proportion of elderly abuse witnessed and the level of social capital.

However, the following limitations can be pointed out. As the association was an ecological one, found between variables calculated for different districts, the effects of confounders were not taken into account. Depending on the way these variables are controlled, this association might disappear. In addition, the amount of data does not seem sufficient. Needless to say, further studies are warranted, including examination of reproducibility of the results using data from larger and more varied communities, and analysis taking confounders into account.

How does social capital influence health?

How is social capital associated with health, or how does it influence health? There are two potential pathways for the association and/or influence[28].

One is the pathway through which the characteristics of individuals in a community may influence their health. It is known that a community with poor social capital has a large proportion of poor people. This means that the association or influence may simply represent the effects of socioeconomic factors on individuals.

For instance, let us divide the subjects into five groups according to equivalent income (total household income divided by the square root of the number of persons in the household). The proportion of those who participated in 'two or more' community organisations was 21.1% in the highest income group, while the corresponding proportion was as low as 9.4% in the lowest income group. Conversely, the proportion of those who participated in no group was high (74.9%) in the lowest income group, and low (53.7%) in the highest income group. As for the norms of reciprocity, as represented by the question, 'Do you think people usually try to help others?', the proportion of subjects who answered 'Yes' was high (33.4%) in the highest income group, and low (21.6%) in the lowest income group. Conversely, the proportion of subjects who answered 'No' was high (15.3%) in the lowest income group, and low (7.4%) in the highest income group[33].

The other potential pathway involves what are known as contextual effects, and is a way of influencing individual health beyond the above-described characteristics of individuals. This is a pathway for effects from the community in which individuals live, independent from their individual characteristics. What influences the health of people in the community through this pathway is community-level social capital in the proper sense of the word. Ichirō Kawachi and Lisa F. Berkman list the following four potential pathways through which this social capital influences health[28].

The first is changes in health behaviour. A community with richer social capital and with good norms is more likely to bring about desirable health behaviour for its members. Similarly, members of a community where voluntary pastimes are actively pursued are more likely to have increased physical exercise because of participating in those activities.

The second pathway is an increase in health services and amenities. The more united residents are, the more likely a community will receive requests for, and opportunities to realise, improvement of parks, gateball courts and other facilities for exercise, provision of health education classes and so on. The unity of a community also promotes protection of a healthy environment by such means as campaigns against pollution.

The third pathway is a psychosocial process. If a community is supported by a feeling of trust, its members will have less psychosocial stress and better mental health. However, this potential pathway of action has been criticised by many for focusing too much on psychological aspects, and for paying little attention to institutional and material aspects[27, 37, 45].

The fourth pathway is the effect of province/state- and local-level policies. Putnam has shown that communities with richer social capital have higher voter turnouts and better performance of various systems, including childcare and healthcare-related facilities[23, 36].

Criticism of social capital

While social capital has attracted the attention of researchers in many fields (international organisations including the World Bank, and domestic organisations including the Japanese Cabinet Office), it has also received criticisms[27]. Major criticisms are outlined below.

Rhetoric or science?

The recent attention paid to social capital is inseparable from the historical background of its rediscovery[22, 25]. Amid the widening gap between rich and poor, the deteriorating sense of personal safety, and the growing emphasis on competition and individualism, many feel uneasy and see problems in the declining norms of mutual support and the breakdown of communities. Initially, the concept and theory of social capital gave us the impression that it might be able to explain these phenomena and improve communities' problem-solving abilities. As such, social capital has attracted a lot of attention as rhetoric, even though it might be a mere hypothesis from a scientific point of view[37, 45]. Michael Woolcock has been quoted as saying, social capital 'risks trying to explain too much with too little'[37].

However, although it has yet to be fully established, examination of social capital using scientific methods has already begun.

Concepts and definitions

The concepts and definitions of social capital have also been the target of many criticisms. One criticism is that social capital has become a buzzword (which is used by different people with different meanings) before a precise definition has been established, due to its interdisciplinary use[22, 27, 37]. Another criticism is that social capital, as a buzzword, attempts to explain what other traditional concepts and terms (such as 'collective efficacy' and 'community competence') can explain, and it has thus caused confusion[26, 37, 46].

Multifactorial, multifaceted concepts and definitions

The factors and facets of social capital included in its concepts and definitions include objective, structural ones, such as the number of community organisations; also functional ones, such as coordinated activities; and subjective, cognitive factors, such as a sense of trust or mutual support.

In addition, while community organisations seem to constitute an objective indicator, different organisations might involve different concepts. For instance, vertical (more traditional) organisations that focus on authority and hierarchical structure, as represented by the Catholic church, might involve a sense of duty or a feeling of smothering, compared to (newer) horizontal organisations, as represented by volunteer groups. For this reason, some have argued that these two types of organisations should be distinguished from each other[23, 27].

Furthermore, a strong sense of solidarity does not always bring good results. Some corporate or organisational crimes occur partly due to solidarity among members. This means that social capital could act negatively. It is not appropriate to emphasise only the positive aspects of social capital.

How should we classify or combine these various aspects of social capital? There is a lot of work to be done on the definition and at the conceptual level, as well as on other levels.

What indicators should be used to measure social capital?

Because the concepts and definitions of social capital include many factors and facets, no consensus has been reached as to what indicators should be used to measure it[22, 40]. A number of questions and measures have been applied to communities in demonstrative studies to date.

For instance in Italy, Putnam used four indicators to calculate a citizen community index, which represents social capital. These indicators included two kinds of voting rates in elections, newspaper subscription rates, and the number of sports and cultural groups per unit of population[23]. On the other hand, Putnam formulated a social capital index comprising a set of fourteen indicators to measure social capital in US states[36]. These indicators included participation in community organisations (whether voluntary or not), the voting rate in presidential elections, a sense of trust in people, and so on. Lochner, Kawachi and Kennedy made a review of similar constructive concepts, in which they note that over 120 questions have been used to measure social capital[26].

There are still many issues to be clarified. For example, if we use the voting rate as an indicator of social capital, is the voting rate itself social capital, or does it represent social capital, or is it a result brought about by social capital?

Conclusion

In this chapter, I have discussed the association between social relationships and health at both an individual level and community or society level. For those whose views have been wholly accustomed to the biomedical model (as was the case with me), the idea that social relationships influence health may well look like an unscientific, lay view, with a wide gap existing between the two.

However, if we do examine ourselves, we realise that most pressured situations, which would place undue stress on our heart, are caused by personal relationship problems or conflicts within other social relationships. Furthermore, most people must know from personal experience that they feel relieved and comforted when they receive emotional support from people close to them. Demonstrative studies supporting these ideas have been accumulating considerably.

In other words, the association between social relationships and health was invisible because we did not attempt to see it; but it does become more apparent if we use appropriate means. Already we can say that the association between social relationships and health at the 'individual level' has been established by evidence from a number of cohort studies. In addition, the association between factors at a 'society level', as represented by social capital, and the health of people who belong to that society seems to exist intuitively and does make an attractive hypothesis, even though this association has not been fully demonstrated. Future research seems to require theoretical studies on social capital, empirical studies on social capital, including refinement of measuring methods, construction of a theoretical hypothesis for the mechanisms by which social capital influences health, and demonstration of the hypothesis based on large-scale data.

Acknowledgment

I am grateful to the 21st Century Center of Excellence Program of the Ministry of Education, Culture, Sports, Science and Technology for its financial support, through the Nihon Fukushi University's project, 'Asian COE: Towards a New Policy Science for Social Wellbeing and Development'.

Literature

1 Kondō, K. (2005), *Kenkō kakusa shakai – nani ga kokoro to kenkō wo mushibamu no ka* (Health Gap Society – what affects our mental and physical health?), Igaku Shoin.
2 Noguchi, Y. (1991), 'Kōreisha no sōsharu sapōto – sono gainen to sokutei (Social support to the elderly – its concept and measurement)', *Shakai rōnen gaku* (Social Gerontology), 34, pp. 37–48.
3 Fukunishi, I. (1997), *Sōsharu sapōto* (Social support), Tokyo: Shibundō.
4 Noguchi, Y. and H. Sugisawa (1998), 'Shakai teki chūtai to kenkō (Social bonds and health)', in H. Orimo (ed), *Shin rōnen gaku* (New Gerontology), Tokyo: University of Tokyo Press, pp. 1343–1348.
5 Stansfeld, S. A. (1999), 'Social support and social cohesion', in M. Marmot and R. G. Wilkinson (eds), *Social Determinants of Health*, Oxford: Oxford University Press, pp. 155–178.
6 House, J. S., K. R. Landis and D. Umberson (1988), 'Social relationships and health', *Science*, 214, pp. 540–545.
7 Ross, C. E., J. Mirowsky and K. Goldsteen (1990), 'The impact of the family on health: the decade in review', *Journal of Marriage and the Family*, 52, pp. 1059–1078.
8 Goldman, N. and Y. Hu (1993), 'Excess mortality among the unmarried: a case study of Japan', *Social Science and Medicine*, 36, pp. 533–546.
9 Baba, Y., K. Kondō and K. Suemori (2003), 'Kekkon to shinri teki kenkō – haikei to shite no shakai keizai teki chii (Marriage and psychological health – socioeconomic status as background', *Kikan kakei keizai kenkyū* (Japanese Journal of Research on Household Economics), 58, pp. 77–85.
10 Kondō, K. (ed.) (2007), 'Kensho "Kenko kakusa syakai" – Kaigo yobou ni muketa syakai ekigakuteki daikibo tyousa.' (Exploring 'Inequalities in Health': A large-scale social epidemiological survey for care preveintion in Japan), Igaku-Shoin.
11 Suemori, K. 'Katei Seikatsu' (Family life). Katsunori Kondō ed. (2007), 'Kensho "Kenko kakusa syakai" – Kaigo yobou ni muketa syakai ekigakuteki daikibo tyousa.' (Exploring 'Inequalities in Health': A large-scale social epidemiological survey for care prevention in Japan), Igaku-Shoin, pp. 75-81.
12 Berkman, L. F. and S. L. Syme (1979), 'Social networks, host resistance, and mortality: a nine-year follow-up study of Alameda County residents', *American Journal of Epidemiology*, 109, pp. 186-203.
13 Kawachi, I., G. A. Colditz, A. Ascherio, E. B. Rimm, E. Giovannucci, M. J. Stampfer and W. C. Willett (1996), 'A prospective study of social networks

in relation to total mortality and cardiovascular disease in men in the USA', *Journal of Epidemiology and Community Health*, 50, pp. 245-251.
14. Seeman, T. E., G. A. Kaplan, L. Knudsen, R. Cohen and J. Guralnik (1987), 'Social network ties and mortality among the elderly in the Alameda County Study', *American Journal of Epidemiology*, 126, pp. 714-723.
15. Vogt, T. M., J. P. Mullooly, D. Ernst, C. R. Pope and J. F. Hollis (1992), 'Social networks as predictors of ischemic heart disease, cancer, stroke and hypertension: incidence, survival and mortality', *Journal of Clinical Epidemiology*, 45, pp. 659-666.
16. Sugisawa, H., J. Liang and X. Li (1994), 'Social networks, social support, and mortality among older people in Japan', *Journal of Gerontology*, 49, pp. S3-13.
17. Okado, J. and T. Hoshi (2002), 'Shakai teki nettowāku ga kōreisha no seimei yogo ni oyobosu eikyō (Effects of social networks on vital prognosis of the elderly)', *Kōsei no shihyō* (Journal of Health and Welfare Statistics), 49, pp. 19-23.
18. Bennett, K. M. (2002), 'Low level social engagement as a precursor of mortality among people in later life', *Age and Aging*, 31, pp. 165-168.
19. Saitō, Y. 'Syakaiteki sapōto' (Social support). K. Kondō (ed.) (2007), 'Kensho "Kenko kakusa syakai" – Kaigo yobou ni muketa syakai ekigakuteki daikibo tyousa.' (Exploring 'Inequalities in Health': A large-scale social epidemiological survey for care prevention in Japan), Igaku-Shoin, pp. 91-97.
20. Yoshii, K., K. Kondō, J. Kuze and K. Higuchi (2005), 'Chiiki zaijū kōreisha no shakai kankei no tokuchō to sono go 2 nenkan no yō kaigo jōtai hassei to no kanrensei (The association between characteristics of social relationships of community-dwelling elderly persons and the occurrence of a state in need of nursing care in the following two years)', *Nihon kōshū eisei zasshi* (Japanese Journal of Public Health), 52, pp. 456-467.
21. Satō, H. (2001), *Enjo to shakai kankei shihon – sōsharu kyapitaru ron no kanōsei* (Aid and social capital: Potentials of the concept of social capital), Chiba: Institute of Developing Economies.
22. Macinko, J. and B. Starfield (2001), 'The utility of social capital in research on health determinants', *The Milbank Quarterly*, 79, pp. 387-427, IV.
23. Putnam, R. D. (1993), *Making Democracy Work*, Princeton: Princeton University Press.
24. Baker, W. E. (2000), *Achieving Success Through Social Capital*, San Francisco: Jossey-Bass, (Translated by Nakajima, Yutaka 2001: Tokyo, Diamond, Inc.).
25. Hawe, P. and A. Shiell (2000), 'Social capital and health promotion: a review', *Social Science and Medicine*, 51, pp. 871-885.
26. Lochner, K., I. Kawachi and B. P. Kennedy (1999), 'Social capital: a guide to its measurement', *Health Place*, 5, pp. 259-270.
26. Whitehead, M. and F. Diderichsen (2001), 'Social capital and health: tiptoeing through the minefield of evidence', *Lancet*, 358, pp. 165-166.
28. Kawachi, I. and L. F. Berkman (2000), 'Social cohesion, social capital, and health', in L. F. Berkman and I. Kawachi (eds), *Social Epidemiology*, New York: Oxford University Press, pp. 174-190.
29. Sampson, R. J., S. W. Raudenbush and F. Earls (1997), 'Neighborhoods and violent crime: a multilevel study of collective efficacy', *Science*, 277, pp. 918-924.

30 Kaneko, I. (2002), *Shinpan komyuniti soryūshon – borantarī na mondai kaiketsu ni muke te* (New edition: community solution – towards voluntary solutions of problems)', Tokyo: Iwanami Shoten.
31 Kreuter, M. W., N. A. Lezin, L. Young and A. N. Koplan (2001), 'Social capital: evaluation implications for community health promotion', *WHO Regional Publications, European Series*, 92, pp. 439-462.
32 Kawachi, I., B. P. Kennedy and R. Glass (1999), 'Social capital and self-rated health: a contextual analysis', *American Journal of Public Health*, 89, pp. 1187-1193.
33 Ichida, Y., G. Yoshikawa, R. Matsuda, K. Kondō, H. Hirai, Y. Saitō, C. Murata, T. Takeda, K. Ishii and M. Nakade (2005), 'Nihon no kōreisha – kaigo yobō ni muketa shakai ekigaku teki daikibo chōsa, 11, Sōsharu kyapitaru to kenkō (The elderly in Japan – a large-scale social epidemiological survey toward prevention of disability, 11, Social capital and health)', *Kōshū Eisei* (Public Health), 69, pp. 914-919.
34 Kawachi, I., B. P. Kennedy, K. Lochner and D. Prothrow-Stith (1997), 'Social capital, income inequality, and mortality', *American Journal of Public Health*, 87, pp. 1491-1498.
35 Veenstra, G. (2002), 'Social capital and health (plus wealth, income inequality and regional health governance', *Social Science and Medicine*, 54, pp. 849-868.
36 Putnam, R. D. (2000), *Bowling Alone: The Collapse and Revival of American Community*, New York: Simon & Schuster.
37 Muntaner, C., J. Lynch and G. D. Smith (2001), 'Social capital, disorganized communities, and the third way: understanding the retreat from structural inequalities in epidemiology and public health', *International Journal of Health Services*, 31, pp. 213-237.
38 Kawachi, I., B. P. Kennedy and R. G. Wilkinson (1999), 'Crime: social disorganization and relative deprivation', *Social Science and Medicine*, 48, pp. 719-739.
39 Kennedy, B. P., I. Kawachi, D. Prothrow-Stith, K. Lochner and V. Gupta (1998), 'Social capital, income inequality, and firearm violent crime', *Social Science and Medicine*, 47, pp. 7-17.
40 Grootaert, C. (1998), 'Social capital: the missing link?', *Social Capital Initiative Working Paper*, No.3, Washington D.C.: The World Bank.
41 Inaba, Y. (2002), *Nihon keizai to shinrai no keizai gaku* (Japanese Economy and Economics of Trust), Tokyo: Tōyō Keizai Shinpō-sha.
42 Lochner, K., E. R. Pamuk, D. Makuc, B. P. Kennedy and I. Kawachi (2001), 'State-level income inequality and individual mortality risk: a prospective, multilevel study', *American Journal of Public Health*, 91, pp. 385-391.
43 Hirai, H. and K. Kondō (2004), 'Chiiki reberu no sōsharu kyapitaru to kōrei sha gyakutai hassei wariai no kanren (The association between community-level social capital and the incidence of elder abuse)', *Nihon Hoken Fukushi Gakkai Dai 17-kai Gakujutsu Shūkai Jiyū Kenkyū Hōkoku Yōshi-shū* (The 17th Conference of Japanese Society of Human Science of Health-Social Services, Abstracts of Independent Study Reports), pp. 26-27.
44 Katō, E., K. Kondō, K. Higuchi and J. Kuze (2004), 'Gyakutai ga utagawareta kōreisha no jōkyō kaizen ni kanren suru yōin – kaigo hoken seido dōnyū zengo no henka (Factors related to improvement of the

situations of elderly persons suspected of experiencing abuse – changes before and after the introduction of nursing care insurance)', *Rōnen shakai kagaku* (Japanese Journal of Gerontology), 25, pp. 482–493.
45 Lynch, J., G. D. Smith, M. Hillemeier, M. Shaw, T. Raghunathan and G. Kaplan (2001), 'Income inequality, the psychosocial environment, and health: comparisons of wealthy nations', *Lancet*, 358, pp. 194–200.
46 Labonte, R. (1999), 'Social capital and community development: practitioner emptor', *Australian and New Zealand Journal of Public Health*, 23, pp. 430–433.

Part III
Research Methods and Ethics

10 Multilevel Analysis of Socioeconomic Factors

Nobuo Nishi

Introduction

Determinants of health include not only individual factors but also social and environmental factors. Social epidemiology attempts to elucidate and develop methods of intervening in these social and environmental factors. Let me take risk factors for ischemic heart disease as an example. In Japan, there has been an emphasis on the significance of personal lifestyle behaviours (such as smoking and physical inactivity) to lifestyle-related diseases (for example, hypertension, hyperlipidemia and diabetes). In contrast, Western countries have recently focused more on the potential role of socioeconomic factors in ischemic heart disease. Studies from these countries include reports of widening disparities in ischemic heart disease mortality related to socioeconomic status[1,2].

Data dealt with in social epidemiology include not only those at the individual level but also those one level above in terms of a hierarchical structure, namely, area-level or occupational-level data. Let us refer to these area (or occupational)-level data as 'group data'. We need to collect and include group data in an analysis.

One example of a study that deals with group data is an 'ecologic study'. This is an effective way of analysing the relationships between different sets of group data. For instance, it is used to analyse links between the average serum total cholesterol level and ischemic heart disease mortality by comparing data from different countries. In an 'ecologic study', however, since analysis is based on group data, analysing individual-level relationships from a group data analysis could lead to wrong inferences. This problem has long been known as an 'ecologic fallacy'[3].

Table 10.1: Types of fallacy in epidemiological studies

Unit of analysis	Level of inference	Type of fallacy
Group	Individual	Ecologic
Group (excluding individual-level variables)	Group	Sociologistic
Individual	Group	Atomistic
Individual (excluding group-level variables)	Individual	Psychologistic

Source: Diez-Roux (1998)[4]. Modified and reproduced with permission from American Public Health Association.

Fallacies in epidemiological studies can be classified into four types, including the 'ecologic fallacy'[4]. Table 10.1 shows the four types, together with the units of analysis and levels of inference. An 'ecologic fallacy' occurs when making individual-level inferences based on results from a group-level analysis. Even when making group-level inferences based on results from a group-level analysis, a 'sociologistic fallacy' may occur if one fails to take into account the effects of individual-level variables which have been excluded from the analysis. The type of fallacy that occurs when making group-level inferences based on results from an individual-level analysis is known as an 'atomistic fallacy'. Even when making individual-level inferences based on results from an individual-level analysis, the 'psychologistic fallacy' may occur if one fails to take into account the effects of group-level variables which have been excluded from the analysis.

In epidemiological studies, it is important to pay attention to the risk of these fallacies in making inferences, and to use the analytical method that matches the level of the subject under observation. Then, if one were to conduct group-level analysis and individual-level analysis at the same time, it would be necessary to use different analytical methods for the different analyses. Out of this necessity, multilevel analysis was developed.

Basics of multilevel analysis

Multilevel analysis is '(i)ntegration of group or macro-level variables into epidemiologic studies in order to incorporate multiple levels of determinants into the study of health outcomes'[5]. It originally developed in the fields of sociology and education.

Figure 10.1: Hierarchical data (of schools as an example)

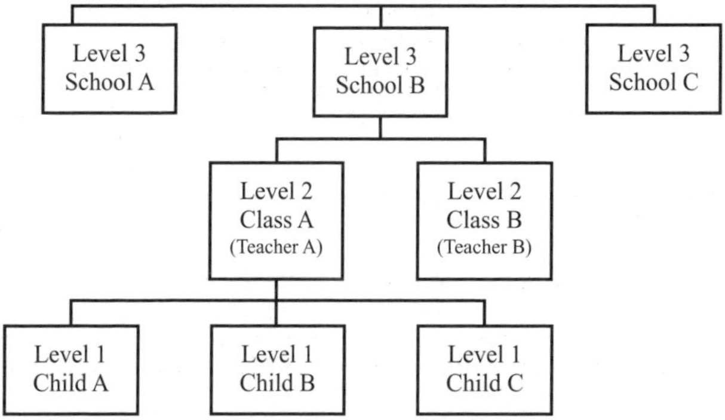

```
┌─────────────┐   ┌─────────────┐   ┌─────────────┐
│   Level 3   │   │   Level 3   │   │   Level 3   │
│  School A   │   │  School B   │   │  School C   │
└─────────────┘   └──────┬──────┘   └─────────────┘
                         │
              ┌──────────┴──────────┐
        ┌─────────────┐      ┌─────────────┐
        │   Level 2   │      │   Level 2   │
        │   Class A   │      │   Class B   │
        │ (Teacher A) │      │ (Teacher B) │
        └──────┬──────┘      └─────────────┘
               │
       ┌───────┼────────┐
 ┌──────────┐ ┌──────────┐ ┌──────────┐
 │ Level 1  │ │ Level 1  │ │ Level 1  │
 │ Child A  │ │ Child B  │ │ Child C  │
 └──────────┘ └──────────┘ └──────────┘
```

Since the 1990s, it has also been widely used in the fields of public health and epidemiology.

Levels of variables on hierarchical levels

As its name implies, multilevel analysis deals with variables on two or more hierarchical levels. Let me take education data as an example. Potential levels of data would be multiple, including children at the individual level, above which would be classes at the group level, above which would come schools (Figure 10.1). Let us simplify this and suppose there are two levels: the micro-level and the macro-level. Epidemiological studies generally analyse variables on the individual level (i.e. micro-level) and the area (or occupational) level (i.e. macro-level). Table 10.2 shows a summary of the levels of variables used in ecological (or 'ecologic') analysis, individual-level analysis and multilevel analysis[6].

Types of variables

Area-level variables can be classified into several types depending on the study subjects and study design. The following are three types based on the structure of variables:
1. Aggregate variables
   An aggregate variable is created by converting the summary statistic of an individual-level variable into a variable (e.g. the proportion of smokers, the median of household income). In an aggregate variable created from an individual-level variable,

Table 10.2: Levels of subjects by types of analysis

	Level of objective variables	Level of explanatory variables	Level of variation	Remarks
Ecological	Group	Group	Group	Not suited for observing interindividual variation
Individual-level	Individual	Individual	Individual	Not suited for observing intergroup variation
Multilevel	Individual	Group and individual	Group and individual	

Source: Table 3-2 from Diez-Roux (2003)[6]. Modified with permission from Oxford University Press.

the issue of multi-colinearity (described below) often occurs.

2. Environmental variables
   An environmental variable is created from observations of the area-level environment (e.g. air pollution level, daylight hours) and not from observations on the individual level.
3. Global variables
   A global variable can be defined on the area level only (e.g. population density, presence/absence of a special bylaw).

Contextual and compositional effects

One of the objectives of multilevel analysis is to elucidate the effects of area-level factors that cannot be detected from an analysis of individual-level factors only. In this regard, let me explain the difference between a contextual effect and a compositional effect.

A contextual effect exists if the effect of an area-level factor cannot be explained solely by one or more individual-level factors. In contrast, a compositional effect is the apparent effect of an area-level factor which seems to exist due to the uneven distribution of one or more individual-level factors in different geographical areas. Suppose, for instance, the incidence of a certain disease is different in different areas. If this is simply because the proportion of people susceptible to that disease is different in different areas, the observed differences in incidence are a compositional effect. If the differences in incidence between the areas cannot be explained solely by the differences in the proportion of susceptible people, and some area-specific factor is likely to exist, then the observed differences in incidence are a contextual effect.

Figure 10.2: Types of contextual effect

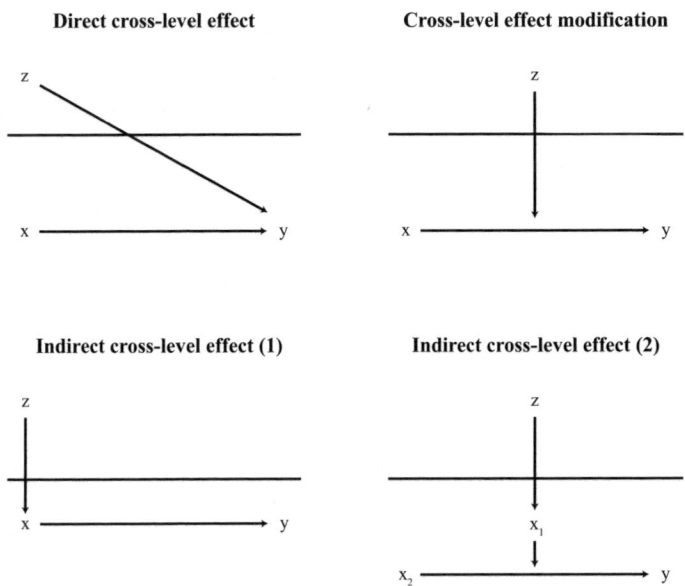

Source: Figure 1 from Blakely & Woodward (2000)[7]. Modified with permission from BMJ Publishing Group.

In multilevel analysis, a contextual effect exists if some effect of an area-level factor remains after adjustment for the effects of individual-level factors.

Types of contextual effects

Blakely and his colleagues categorised contextual effects into three types: 'direct cross-level effects', 'cross-level effect modifications' and 'indirect cross-level effects' (Figure 10.2)[7].

1. Direct cross-level effects
   A direct cross-level effect is the direct effect of area-level exposure variable z on individual-level consequential variable y that is independent of the effect of individual-level exposure variable x on consequential variable y.
2. Cross-level effect modifications
   A cross-level effect modification is the modification by area-level exposure variable z of the effect of individual-

level exposure variable x on individual-level consequential variable y.
3. Indirect cross-level effects
Indirect cross-level effects occur in two different ways. First, area-level exposure variable z has an effect on individual-level exposure variable x. Second, when individual-level exposure variable x_1 modifies the effect of individual-level exposure variable x_2 on individual-level consequential variable y, the effect of area-level exposure variable z on individual-level exposure variable x_1 is an indirect cross-level effect.

Intraclass correlation

Social epidemiology focuses on effects at the area level, which is one level above the individual level. Therefore, social epidemiology focuses on contextual effects. When assessing contextual effects in a multilevel analysis, regression coefficients are frequently used as indicators of association. In contrast, intraclass correlations, which are used to assess contextual effects based on variation, are seldom used[8]. Below I explain intraclass correlations using a multilevel regression analysis model.

An intraclass correlation can be expressed by the following simple formula:

Interclass variance / (intraclass variance + interclass variance)

In social epidemiology, interclass variance and intraclass variance generally mean inter-area variance and intra-area variance, respectively. In terms of an individual-level objective variable, if individuals from the same area are more similar to each other than to those from another area, the intraclass variance is relatively small compared to the interclass variance, and the intraclass correlation is large.

No clear standard has been established with regard to the level of intraclass correlation above which a contextual effect should be found to exist. Related to this, in their review on intraclass correlation, Merlo and colleagues propose an intraclass correlation of 8% based on virtual data in which the objective variable is systolic blood pressure[8].

The intraclass correlation can be calculated using the above formula in a random intercept model, but cannot be calculated easily in a random slope model or if the objective variable is not normally distributed (for instance, if the objective variable is binary)[9, 10].

*Figure 10.3: Association between age and blood pressure level –
Example 1 (total number)*

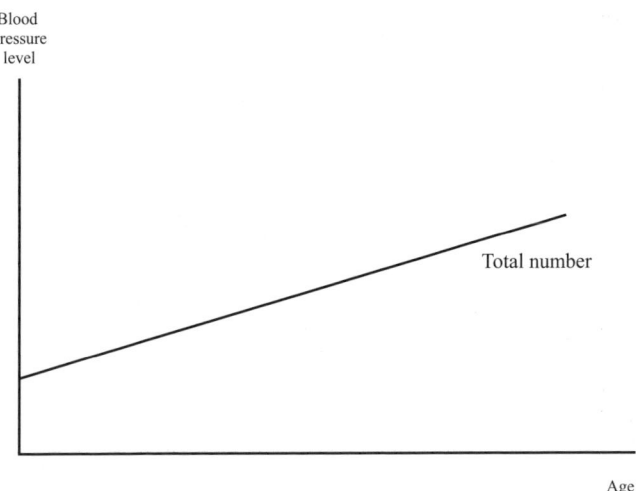

Theory of multilevel analysis

Below I describe the use of conventional analysis models on hierarchical data, including multiple regression analysis, logistic regression analysis, and multilevel analysis. First, let me give a conceptual explanation of the significance of multilevel analysis.

Significance of multilevel analysis

Using the association between age and blood pressure level as an example, I provide a conceptual explanation of the significance of using multilevel analysis, instead of individual-level analysis, on hierarchical data. For this purpose, I use a linear regression model in which blood pressure levels increase simply with age, without regard for all other factors.

Figure 10.3 shows the association between age and blood pressure level for the total number of both men and women. Blood pressure (BP) levels can be calculated by the following equation:

$$BP = \beta_0 + \beta_1 age$$

where β_0 and β_1 are the coefficients representing intercept and slope, respectively.

Figure 10.4-1: Association between age and blood pressure level – Example 2 (by sex)

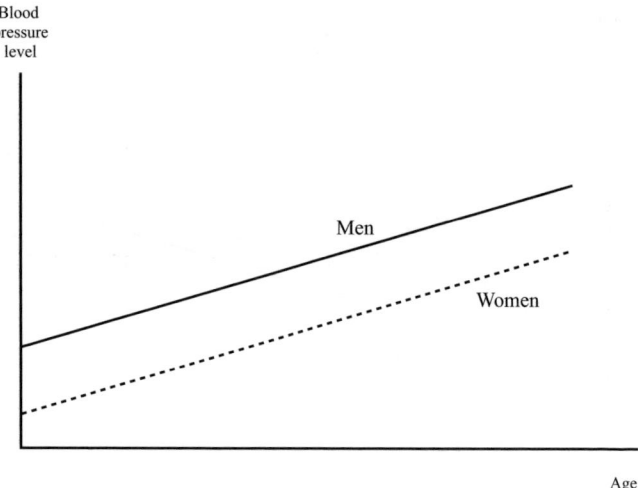

If women generally have higher BP levels than men at a certain level, the associations between age and BP level for men and women will look like Figure 10.4-1. BP levels can be calculated with the following equation:

$$BP = \beta_0 + \beta_1 age + \beta_2 sex$$

where β_2 is the coefficient representing the difference between men and women.

Similarly to the gender difference in BP, if BP levels vary in different areas at certain levels, the associations between age and BP level for different areas will look like Figure 10.4-2. BP levels can be calculated with the following equation:

$$BP = \beta_0 + \beta_1 age + \beta_2 area$$

where β_2 is the coefficient representing the differences among the areas. If the number of areas is large, however, the area term will have to be represented by a dummy variable of one less than the number of the areas, resulting in reduced statistical power.

If women generally have higher BP levels than men by a certain rate, the associations between age and BP level for men and women will look like Figure 10.5-1. BP levels can be calculated with the following equation:

Figure 10.4-2: Association between age and blood pressure level – Example 2 (by area)

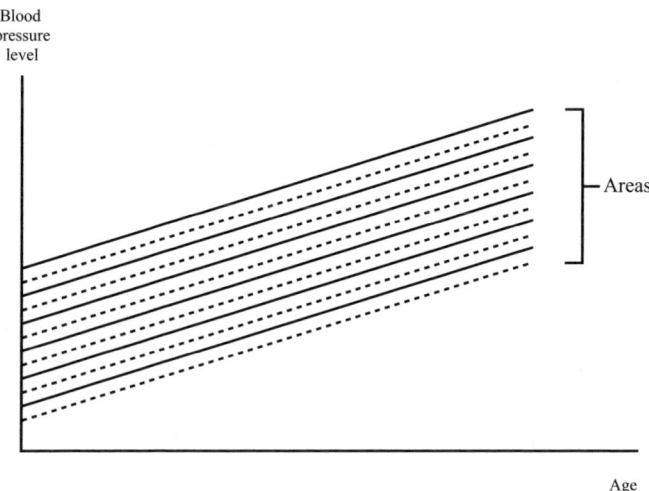

$$BP = \beta_0 + \beta_1 age + \beta_2 sex + \beta_3 age*sex$$

where β_3 is the coefficient representing the interaction between age and sex.

If, similar to the sexual difference in BP, BP levels differ in different areas by certain rates, the associations between age and BP level for different areas will look like Figure 10.5-2. BP levels can be calculated with the following equation:

$$BP = \beta_0 + \beta_1 age + \beta_2 area + \beta_3 age*area$$

where β_3 is the coefficient representing the interaction between age and area. If the number of areas is large, however, the main effect term and the interaction term will each have to be represented by a dummy variable of one less than the number of the areas, resulting in extremely reduced statistical power.

As shown in Figures 10.4-2 and 10.5-2, if, due to a large number of areas, the main effect term and the interaction term have to each be represented by a dummy variable of one less than the number of the areas, the statistical power will be extremely reduced. In order to solve this problem, multilevel analysis allows these many dummy variables to be represented by only one variable, by focusing on the intercept and the slope in Figure 10.4-2 and Figure

Figure 10.5-1: Association between age and blood pressure level – Example 3 (by sex)

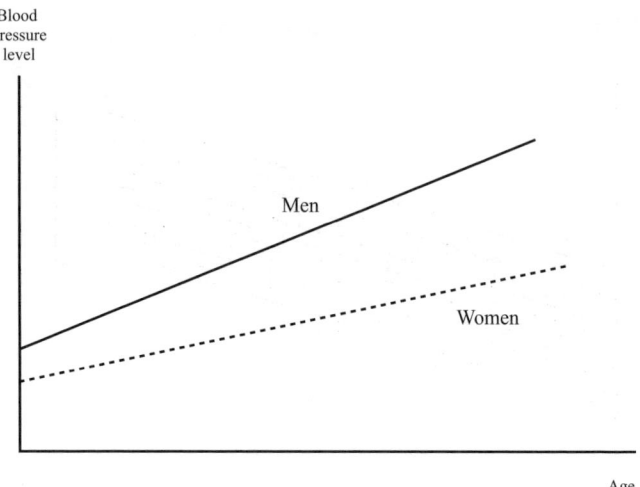

10.5-2, respectively. Specifically, the models represented by Figure 10.4-2 and that by Figure 10.5-2 are a random intercept model and a random slope model, respectively, in multilevel analysis, and are described below.

Conventional analysis models

Let me discuss how to analyse data containing both individual-level and area-level variables using a conventional analysis model, that is, a multiple regression analysis that assumes fixed effects only. Suppose that for the ith person of the jth group, Y_{ij} is the objective variable, x_{ij} is the individual-level explanatory variable, and z_j is the area-level explanatory variable. The regression formula would be:

$$Y_{ij} = \beta_0 + \beta_1 x_{ij} + \beta_2 z_{ij} + R_{ij} \tag{1}$$

where β_0 is the intercept, β_1 and β_2 are the coefficients of individual-level variable x and area-level variable z, and R is the residual error (or accidental error), whose average is zero. Formula (1) includes the main effects only, namely, individual-level variable x and area-level variable z, but could also include the interaction (between these levels), $z_{ij} x_{ij}$.

Figure 10.5-2: Association between age and blood pressure level – Example 3 (by area)

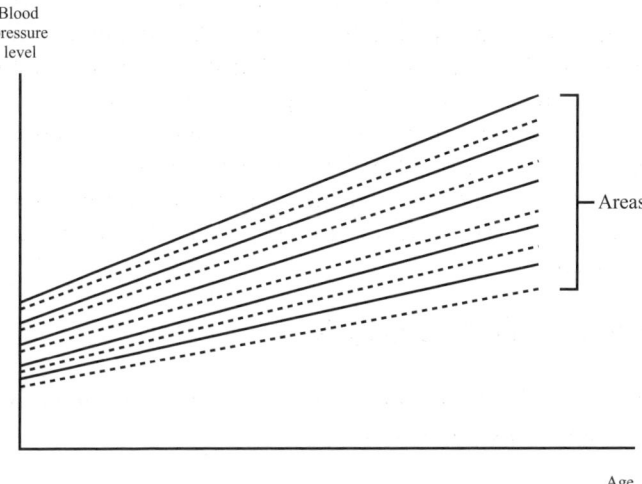

Because this conventional model is based on fixed effects, it assumes that each person is independent of each other. However, if any contextual effect exists in hierarchical data, it is not appropriate to assume that everyone is independent of each other, regardless of which group they belong to. This is why multilevel analysis models were developed.

Multilevel analysis models

There are several types of multilevel analysis models, including multilevel models, random coefficient models, and hierarchical linear models. Mathematically, they are all similar and are characterised by their assumption of random effects as well as fixed effects. Based on the commentary by Snijders and Bosker[10], I outline below the random intercept model and the random slope model that are based on the hierarchical linear model.

As stated above, if any contextual effect exists in hierarchical data, it is not appropriate to assume that everyone is independent of each other, regardless of which group they belong to. Thus, we assume that formula (1) holds for each group. The following regression formula is suggested for the jth group:

$$Y_{ij} = \beta_0 + \beta_1 x_{ij} + \beta_2 z_j + R_{ij} \tag{2}$$

where β_{0j} and β_{1j} are unique coefficients for the jth group. The distributions of the fixed effects and of the random effects are fitted to the distributions of the coefficients of each group. In the random intercept model, the intercept of the regression formula, β_{0j}, is assumed to distribute randomly. In the random slope model, the slope, β_{1j}, is assumed to distribute randomly. It is understood that the random intercept model and the random slope model correspond to direct cross-level effect and cross-level effect modification, respectively[7].

Practice of multilevel analysis

Based on the theory of multilevel analysis, below I summarise the issues requiring consideration.

Points to remember in multilevel analysis

1. Setting an appropriate area level
   It is important to make an appropriate choice of which area level should be focused on, as this influences the individual-level objective variable. For instance, if a household survey is conducted to find information on personal lifestyles, at the area level, the subjects' personal lifestyles are likely to be influenced by their households more than by their areas.
2. Choosing area-level variables
   As described above, area-level variables include aggregate, environmental and global variables and others. Sometimes, however, appropriate data are not available. It is necessary to consider, from the planning stage of the study, what area-level data should be included as well as the sampling method.
3. Confounding and multi-colinearity
   In the association between an area-level explanatory variable and an area-level objective variable, if an individual-level factor is a confounder for this association, and if no variable is included in the model to represent the individual-level factor, then a strong apparent contextual effect may be detected. Even if a variable is included in the model to represent the individual-level factor, and if the area-level explanatory variable is calculated based on one or more individual-level variables (i.e.

if the area-level explanatory variable is an aggregate variable), special attention must be paid to the issue of multi-colinearity.

Application of multilevel analysis

While I have thus far described multilevel analysis based on the individual and area levels, multilevel analysis can be applied to the following cases as well:

1. Cross-classification

    A multilevel analysis can deal with, on the macro-level, occupational communities as well as geographical areas. Multilevel analyses conducted in the field of education, for instance, have taken into account the fact that one school is attended by students from more than one area and that students from the same area attend different schools, unless the school district is restricted to a certain area. Multilevel analysis can simultaneously deal with and analyse these cases, where more than one macro-level variable exists for one person on the individual level.

2. Repeated measurements

    Individuals are not always treated as a micro-level factor; in some cases, they are treated as a macro-level factor. If a certain test is repeated on the same subjects, the results from the repeated tests are influenced considerably by each subject and not by any other subject. Therefore, it is appropriate to conduct a multilevel analysis by treating the test times and the subjects as a micro-level factor and a macro-level factor, respectively. Multilevel analysis has the advantage of allowing analysis even if a data set does not contain results from all test times and even if different subjects had tests at different times. Types of analysis in which this analytical method is used include longitudinal data analysis and growth curve analysis.

3. Meta-analysis

    Meta-analysis is 'a research method that systematically collects results of previous studies on a certain problem, evaluates them qualitatively and synthesizes them quantitatively, whereby each study's results form a unit of a research area'[11]. Meta-analysis can be regarded as a type of multilevel analysis, since each subject of the meta-analysis is an aggregate of personal data. As such, meta-analysis is possible even if the statistics available from the macro-level literature are limited to the effect size, and its standard error is calculated from the micro-level personal data.

Major software products

Below I mention two major software products developed exclusively for multilevel analysis.
1. MLwiN (*http://www.cmm.bristol.ac.uk/*)
   The MLwiN software was developed by Goldstein and his colleagues who participated in the Multilevel Models Project of the Institute of Education, University of London[12]. It meets the needs of multilevel analysis very flexibly. Visit the above website for more information (user manuals are also available).
2. HLM6 (*http://www.ssicentral.com/*)
   The HLM6 software was developed by Bryk and his colleagues. It is easy to use for students as well as researchers. Their website address is shown above.

Of the multipurpose statistical software products, SAS most adequately meets the various needs of multilevel analysis. If the objective variable is continuous data or discrete data, PROC MIXED or PROC NLMIXED should be used, respectively.

An example of multilevel analysis: a Finnish study

Below I describe an example of a study that uses multilevel analysis. The study uses mortality as an indicator, pointing out the results of a previous study which suggested that the effects of area-level variables tend to be more easily observed in subjective indicators, such as self-reported health level, than in objective indicators of health[13]. The original report focuses on alcohol-related diseases and conducts an analysis of causes of death. However, I would like to limit my discussion to the analysis of total mortality and would like to focus on the methods and results as an example of multilevel analysis.

Subjects and methods

1. Study population and death survey
   The study population consisted of 251,509 men aged 25 years and over who lived in the Helsinki Metropolitan area at the time of the 1990 national census. In the total study population,

those aged over 64 years, those who had primary education only, and unskilled manual workers accounted for 11.5%, 36.5% and 14.1%, respectively.

Using personal ID numbers, a link was made by Statistics Finland between the death records for 1991–1995 and data on the study population. Of those who were included in the death records, only about 0.5% could not be identified in the 1990 census data. The study population was followed for a total of 1,220,000 person years and included 14,878 deaths.

2. Individual-level variables

   The following five individual-level socio-demographic variables were used in the study, based on the census data:

   a. Education

      Based on their highest completed educational degree or certificate, the subjects were classified into the categories of 'primary', 'secondary' and 'tertiary-educated'. The secondary category was further divided into 'lower secondary' and 'higher secondary'. In total, four categories were used.

   b. Occupation-based social class

      The subjects were divided into five categories: 'upper white collar', 'lower white collar', 'skilled manual', 'unskilled manual', and 'other' (including farmers, other self-employed, and those whose social class was not known). Unemployed and retired people were classified according to their previous occupations. Those taking care of a household were categorised according to the occupation of the head of the household.

   c. Housing tenure

      Housing tenure was classified as 'owner occupied' or 'other'.

   d. Housing density

      Housing density was assessed in terms of living space per person and categorised into three groups: 'spacious', 'intermediate' and 'crowded'.

   e. Living arrangements

      Living arrangements were classified into two categories: 'living with a partner' (married or cohabiting) or 'living without a partner'.

      For some of these variables, data was missing (unknown) for 2-3% of the total study population. For occupation-based social class and housing tenure, missing data were allocated

into the 'other' categories, and for housing density, put into the 'intermediate' category. Because of the small share of missing values, their allocation had a negligible effect on the results.
3. Area-level variables
Definition of the Helsinki Metropolitan area was based on the administrative area divisions of municipalities. Some smaller areas were merged to obtain areas that were comparable to other areas in terms of size and number of deaths. Areas that were geographically and physically different or diverse in their socio-demographic structure were not merged. Small areas that did not have neighbouring areas that could be merged together, as well as military and campus areas were excluded from this study (five areas). The final area division used in this study consisted of 55 areas, with a population varying from 3,699 to 26,401 (mean = 14,635).

The area variables represented three factors: socioeconomic structure, demographic structure and social cohesion. The authors experimented with several variables for each factor and selected those that had the strongest associations with age-adjusted mortality at the area level. In addition, the authors confirmed that inclusion of any additional area variables was not associated with area mortality in a statistically significant way. The following variables were used in the analysis:

a. Proportion of manual workers
The proportion of manual workers was chosen as the variable for socioeconomic structure. The proportion of male manual workers aged 15–64 years in each area was used.

b. Proportion of people over 60 years old
The proportion of men over 60 years old was chosen as the variable for demographic structure. The proportion of people over 60 years old (both men and women) in each area was used.

c. Social cohesion
Social cohesion was measured by a standardised score calculated from the following three indicators:
- The proportion of men over 15 years old living with a partner at the time of the 1990 census
- The voting percentage in the municipal elections in 1988
- The proportion of men over 15 years old at the time of the 1990 census who did not live in the same area at the time of the 1985 census

These three indicators measured adherence to traditional forms of living arrangements, participation in politics and residential stability, respectively. In an exploratory factor analysis of the data, these three indicators loaded strongly on the same factor.

All area-level variables were measured in four quartiles. For social cohesion, the two middle quartiles were combined into one category. The data were obtained from the municipal statistical authorities and census data aggregated over areas.

4. Statistical methods

Using SAS macro GLIMMIX, a multilevel analysis was conducted based on a random intercept model. In the models the authors used a Poisson distribution assumption, a log link and the logarithm of person years as an offset. In these data, maximum likelihood and restricted maximum likelihood estimation led to substantively similar parameter estimates and confidence intervals; the authors thus used maximum likelihood methods that allow for deviance tests of fixed effects. The analyses were carried out separately for 25–64 year-old men and over 64 year-old men because these age groups vary considerably in their attachment to the labour market and cause of death structure. Within the two broad age groups, age was adjusted for in five-year age groups.

The parameters of the models are presented as 'mortality risk ratios', with those in the reference group having a mortality risk ratio of 1. The mortality risk ratio has the advantage of allowing a straightforward percentage interpretation, for example, a group with a ratio of 1.25 has a 25% higher mortality than the reference group. The authors also calculated average relative deviations, which are statistics representing the variation in mortality between the 55 areas. The average relative deviation shows by how many per cent on average the mortality rate of a given area differs from the total mortality rate.

Results

1. Mortality risk ratios

The mortality risk ratio for the area of highest mortality in relation to the area of lowest mortality was 2.88 among 25–64 year-old men. Table 10.3-1 and Table 10.3-2 show the effects of all area- and individual-level variables on total mortality for the 25–64 year-olds and the over 64 year-olds, respectively.

Table 10.3-1: Age-adjusted mortality and mortality risk ratios by area-level and individual-level variables (25–64 year olds)

	Proportion of deaths	Age-adjusted mortality[a]	Mortality risk ratio				
			Model 1	Model 2	Model 3	Model 4	95% CI
Number of deaths	6,461	589					
Area-level variables							
Proportion of manual workers (%)							
10.2–26.5	20.9	478.2	1.00	1.00		1.00	
26.6–38.9	23.0	521.6	1.14	1.25		1.08	0.99–1.17
39.0–45.3	30.6	657.1	1.39	1.38		1.12	1.03–1.23
45.4–64.0	25.4	723.7	1.58	1.58		1.19	1.10–1.30
Proportion of over 60 year olds (%)							
6.0–9.3	21.3	529.8	1.00	1.00		1.00	
9.4–13.4	23.6	559.1	1.05	0.98		0.98	0.91–1.06
13.5–22.1	24.9	556.1	1.05	1.15		1.06	0.98–1.14
22.2–31.2	30.1	725.5	1.35	1.28		1.08	1.00–1.17
Social cohesion							
High	19.5	456.5	0.77	0.94		1.04	0.96–1.13
Intermediate	49.0	576.1	1.00	1.00		1.00	
Low	31.5	754.2	1.31	1.24		1.11	1.04–1.19
Individual-level variables							
Education							
Tertiary	12.0	305.1	1.00		1.00	1.00	
Higher secondary	12.6	447.4	1.46		1.24	1.24	1.01–1.38
Lower secondary	18.6	661.8	2.19		1.48	1.47	1.32–1.65
Primary	56.9	797.1	2.54		1.59	1.58	1.43–1.75

	Proportion of deaths	Age-adjusted mortality*	Mortality risk ratio			
			Model 1	Model 2	Model 3	Model 4	95% CI
Occupation-based social class							
Upper white collar	16.3	329.6	1.00		1.00	1.00	
Lower white collar	18.2	501.3	1.52		1.12	1.11	1.01–1.22
Skilled manual	30.9	765.5	2.28		1.36	1.35	1.23–1.49
Unskilled manual	23.0	936.3	2.72		1.46	1.45	1.31–1.61
Other	11.6	649.3	1.97		1.39	1.38	1.25–1.54
Housing tenure							
Owner-occupied	53.4	437.1	1.00		1.00	1.00	
Other	46.6	985.2	2.17		1.59	1.58	1.49–1.66
Housing density							
Spacious	34.2	503.5	1.00		1.00	1.00	
Intermediate	56.4	672.6	1.32		1.12	1.12	1.05–1.18
Crowded	9.4	809.4	1.45		1.25	1.22	1.11–1.34
Living arrangements							
With partner	58.1	445.1	1.00		1.00	1.00	
Without partner	41.9	1,064.9	2.30		1.94	1.92	1.82–2.03

Note. a: per 100,000 persons

Source: Table 1 from Martikainen, Kauppinen & Valkonen (2003)[13]. Modified with permission from BMJ Publishing Group.

Table 10.3-2: Age-adjusted mortality and mortality risk ratios by area-level and individual-level variables (over 64 year olds)

	Proportion of deaths	Age-adjusted mortality[a]	Mortality risk ratio				
			Model 1	Model 2	Model 3	Model 4	95% CI
Number of deaths	6,461	589					
Area-level variables							
Proportion of manual workers (%)							
10.2–26.5	29.3	6,018.8	1.00	1.00		1.00	
26.6–38.9	23.0	6,767.8	1.11	1.13		1.04	0.97–1.11
39.0–45.3	27.7	7,313.2	1.20	1.24		1.09	1.01–1.17
45.4–64.0	20.0	7,827.9	1.29	1.30		1.10	1.02–1.19
Proportion of over 60 year olds (%)							
6.0–9.3	12.5	7,063.8	1.00	1.00		1.00	
9.4–13.4	18.0	6,769.8	0.95	0.93		0.94	0.86–1.02
13.5–22.1	29.1	6,811.2	0.96	1.03		1.01	0.93–1.09
22.2–31.2	40.4	6,893.5	0.98	1.01		0.99	0.92–1.07
Social cohesion							
High	22.6	6,248.3	0.88	0.98		0.98	0.93–1.07
Intermediate	46.6	7,146.5	1.00	1.00		1.00	
Low	30.8	7,020.4	1.00	1.00		0.95	0.90–1.01
Individual-level variables							
Education							
Tertiary	17.0	5,325.2	1.00		1.00	1.00	
Higher secondary	10.3	6,351.7	1.17		1.09	1.08	0.99–1.19
Lower secondary	9.5	6,802.1	1.26		1.10	1.09	0.99–1.21
Primary	63.2	7,583.9	1.39		1.15	1.14	1.05–1.23

	Proportion of deaths	Age-adjusted mortality[a]	Mortality risk ratio				
			Model 1	Model 2	Model 3	Model 4	95% CI
Occupation-based social class							
Upper white collar	20.8	5,556.2	1.00		1.00	1.00	
Lower white collar	21.5	6,736.8	1.19		1.03	1.02	0.95–1.11
Skilled manual	35.2	7,474.7	1.30		1.02	1.01	0.93–1.10
Unskilled manual	11.4	8,115.9	1.44		1.05	1.04	0.95–1.15
Other	11.1	7,332.2	1.30		1.08	1.07	0.98–1.17
Housing tenure							
Owner-occupied	73.1	6,339.3	1.00		1.00	1.00	
Other	26.9	8,765.3	1.37		1.18	1.18	1.12–1.24
Housing density							
Spacious	49.0	5,811.5	1.00		1.00	1.00	
Intermediate	44.4	8,184.4	1.39		1.29	1.28	1.22–1.35
Crowded	6.6	9,459.9	1.60		1.55	1.55	1.42–1.70
Living arrangements							
With partner	64.2	6,301.5	1.00		1.00	1.00	
Without partner	35.8	8,437.7	1.31		1.28	1.28	1.22–1.34

Note. a: per 100,000 persons
Source: Table 1 from Martikainen, Kauppinen & Valkonen (2003)[13]. Modified with permission from BMJ Publishing Group.

For the 25–64 year age group, high mortality is observed in areas that are characterised by a high proportion of over 60 year-olds, a high proportion of manual workers, and low social cohesion. Of the individual-level variables analysed, low education, low occupation-based social class, non-ownership of housing, living in crowded accommodation, and not living with a partner are related to high mortality. Overall, the associations of individual-level variables on total mortality are larger than those of area-level variables.

When all area-level variables are entered to the model simultaneously (model 2), the proportion of manual workers shows the strongest association with mortality, while social cohesion considerably attenuates mortality risk ratios. When entering all individual-level variables to the model simultaneously (model 3), all effects are attenuated. However, those with low education, low occupation-based social class, and non-ownership of housing have mortality risk ratios in the region of about 1.5, and those living without a partner have a mortality risk ratio of almost 2.

When both area- and individual-level variables are entered to the multilevel model simultaneously, the effects of area-level variables are further attenuated, while the effects of individual-level variables remain almost unchanged. Of the area-level variables, the proportion of manual workers has the strongest association with total mortality (mortality risk ratio 1.19).

Among the over 64 year-olds, all the effects of area- and individual-level variables on mortality are weaker than among the 25–64 year-olds, with the exception of housing density. Furthermore, when both area- and individual-level variables are entered to the multilevel model simultaneously, all the effects of area-level variables are insignificant, with the exception of a weak effect of the proportion of manual workers. Of the individual-level variables, the effects of housing density and living arrangements remain strong.

2. Area variation measured in terms of average relative deviation

The total area variation in age-adjusted mortality for the 25–64 year-olds, measured in terms of the average relative deviation for all the 55 areas, is 16.6%. In other words, on average the age-adjusted mortality rate of an area differs by 16.6% from the age-adjusted total mortality rate. The corresponding figure is 8.1% for the over 64 year-olds (Table 10.4). In both broad

Table 10.4: *The effects of adjustments for area- and individual-level variables on the average relative deviation in area-level mortality*

		Average relative deviation (%)		
	Only age adjusted	All area-level variables adjusted	All individual-level variables adjusted	All variables adjusted
25–64 year olds	16.6	3.7	4.1	0.3
Over 64 year olds	8.1	1.6	2.6	0.8

Source: Table 2 from Martikainen, Kauppinen & Valkonen (2003)[13]. Modified with permission from BMJ Publishing Group.

age groups, about 80% of the average deviation is accounted for by the three area-level variables, or about 70% by all the individual-level variables, and more than 90% of the average deviation is accounted for by area- and individual-level variables entered to the multilevel model simultaneously.

3. Interactions between area- and individual-level variables
   The authors studied interactions between area-level and individual-level variables to assess whether the effects of individual-level socioeconomic factors on mortality are different in areas with different socioeconomic structure and social cohesion. The interactions are presented in terms of age-adjusted death rates, but similar results are obtained with mortality risk ratios. Individual-level occupation-based social class and education are collapsed into two groups to guarantee adequate numbers of deaths for each combination of the interaction. Specifically, for occupation-based social class, the 'other' category has been excluded, and the subjects are classified as manual workers and white collar workers; and for education, the subjects are classified as primary/lower secondary-educated and higher secondary/tertiary-educated. Within the confines of random variation, the age-adjusted curves are parallel among the 25–64 year-olds and thus indicate little additive interaction between area- and individual-level variables (Figure 10.6). For the over 64 year-olds, interactions between education and area-level variables are quite strong, but inconsistent for the proportion of manual workers (Figure 10.7). Specifically, those with low education have high mortality in areas of both high and low proportions of manual workers, but in areas with average

Figure 10.6: Age-adjusted mortality rates by area- and individual-level variables (25-64 year-olds)

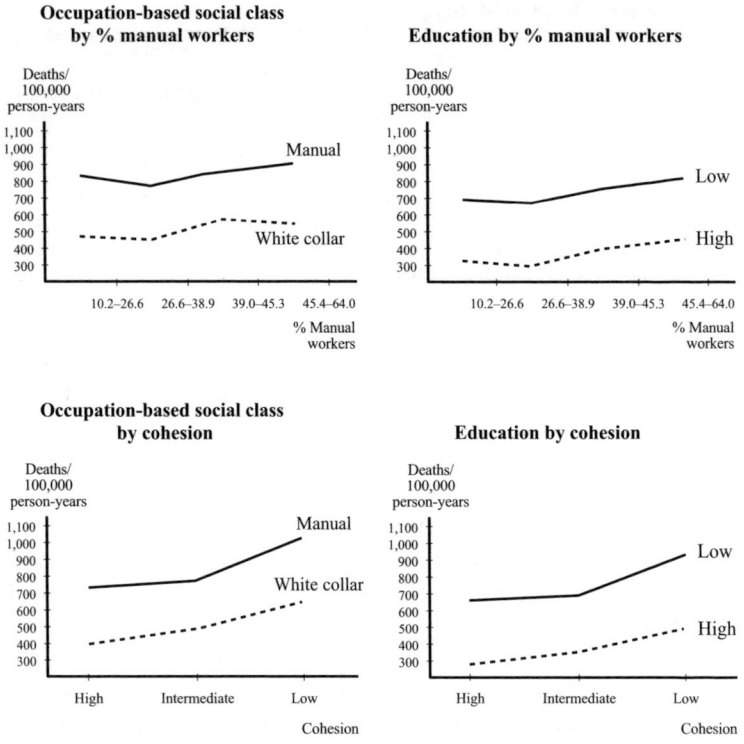

Source: Figure 1 from Martikainen, Kauppinen & Valkonen (2003)[13]. Modified with permission from BMJ Publishing Group.

levels of manual workers the effect of education is small. With regards to social cohesion, those with low education have increased mortality in areas of high cohesion, but this excess is negligible in areas of low cohesion.

Methodological considerations

All analyses of the relative contribution of area-level and individual-level variables on mortality and health status may be compromised by inadequate measurement at both levels. In particular, unaccounted individual-level variability and selective residential migration cannot be excluded as an explanation for the observed effects

Figure 10.7: Age-adjusted mortality rates by area- and individual-level variables (over 64 year-olds)

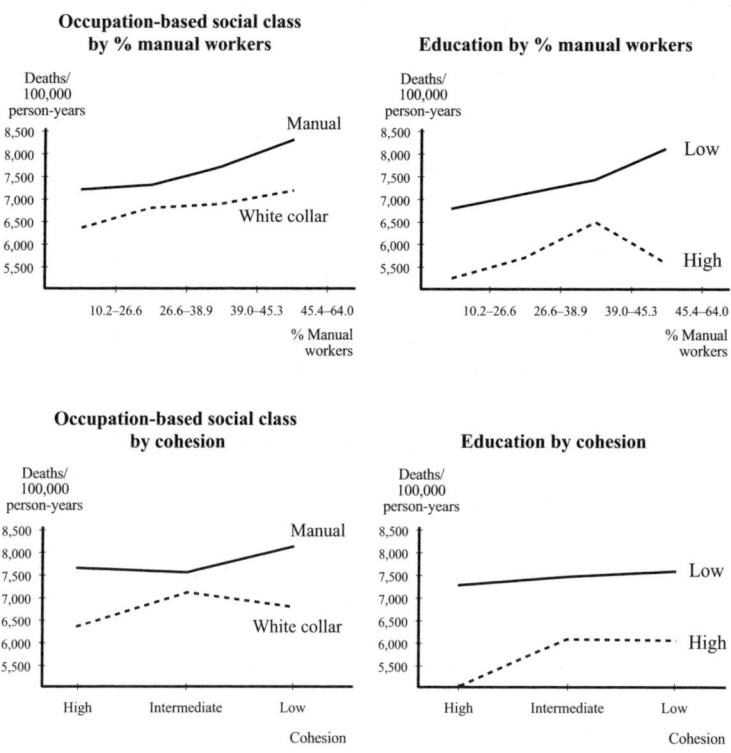

Source: Figure 2 from Martikainen, Kauppinen & Valkonen (2003)[13]. Modified with permission from BMJ Publishing Group.

of area-level variables. This possibility is particularly potent for the several studies that have only been able to adjust for a single socioeconomic confounder at the individual level. However, in the present study with good adjustment for several individual sociodemographic factors, the observed effects of area-level variables on mortality may be taken as good evidence for a modest causal relation of area-level factors on mortality.

It could be argued that it is difficult to observe robust effects of area-level variables because measures of area characteristics are inadequate. In the present study, the authors only used compositional variables (area-level variables that can be obtained by aggregating individual-level variables over areas), rather than integral variables (area-level variables that can only be measured at the area level and have no meaningful parallel at the individual level, for example, quality of roads). However, the compositional variables used in the study are not aggregated within the study population, but are aggregates of the total population or of the population of men aged 15 years and over living in the study areas. It is thus unlikely that inadequate measurement compromised the study results. This is also obvious from the fact that, of the total observed area variation between the 55 areas, about 80% can be accounted for by the area-level variables (about 90% of area variation is accounted for by area- and individual-level variables). Thus, any unaccounted for part of the observed area variation is small.

A possible drawback of the present analysis or, ultimately, any analyses of the effects of area-level variables on health may be that the area levels used are not appropriate for analysing the area-level effects. Further studies are warranted to analyse the effects of area-level variables using different area units, both larger and smaller than those used in the present study. Such analyses may be helpful in some way for elucidating the processes influencing people's health, such as amenities and administrative services in larger area units and control of deviant behaviour in smaller area units.

An example of multilevel analysis: a Japanese study

In Japan, too, several studies have been conducted using multilevel analysis. Since a full account has been given in Chapter 3 of the report by Shibuya and his colleagues[14], below I provide a summary of the work of Fukuda and his colleagues[15], which, similarly to Shibuya's report, uses data from the Comprehensive Survey of Living Conditions of the People on Health and Welfare.

1. Background
   Little is known about the socioeconomic differences in health-related behaviours in Japan. The present study was performed to elucidate the effects of individual and regional socioeconomic factors on selected health risk behaviours among Japanese adults, with a particular focus on regional variations.
2. Methods
   In a nationally representative sample of 25–59 year-olds (20,030 men and 21,076 women), the relationships between six risk behaviours (*i.e.* current smoking, excessive alcohol consumption, poor dietary habits, physical inactivity, stress and non-attendance of health check-ups), individual socio-

economic factors (*i.e.* age, marital status, occupation and household income) and regional (N = 60) socioeconomic factors (per capita income and unemployment rate) were examined by multilevel analysis.

3. Results

Of the individual socioeconomic factors, divorce, employment (as opposed to being housewives) among women, lower occupational class and lower household income were generally associated with a higher likelihood of risk behaviour. The degrees of regional variation in risk behaviour and the influence of regional indicators were greater for women than for men: higher per capita income was significantly associated with current smoking, excessive alcohol consumption, stress and non-attendance of health check-ups among women.

4. Conclusion

Individual lower socioeconomic status was a substantial predictor of risk behaviour in both sexes, while a marked influence of the regional socioeconomic status was observed only for women. The accumulation of risk behaviours in individuals with lower socioeconomic status and among women in areas with higher income, reflecting an urban context, may contribute to their higher mortality rates.

5. Supplement

As described in the Results section, the regional variations in risk behaviours were greater for women than men. The intraclass correlations for current smoking, excessive alcohol consumption, physical inactivity, poor dietary habits, stress and non-attendance of health check-ups were 8.0%, 7.7%, 0.0%, 1.1%, 1.6% and 8.0%, respectively, for men and 26.1%, 11.4%, 2.6%, 8.8%, 2.1% and 11.8%, respectively, among women. Thus, for all health risk behaviours, the intraclass correlations were greater for women than men. These intraclass correlations also show considerable differences in regional variation among different health risk behaviours.

Conclusion

Previous epidemiological studies have mainly used individual-level data, such as personal characteristics (e.g. sex, age), lifestyles and, more recently, genotypes. Most of the (small number of) studies which do use area-level data have attempted to fit the data into a conventional analytical model. Despite its original nature as a science studying human populations, epidemiology has tended to overemphasise individuals.

Countermeasures against lifestyle-related diseases must include intervention not only among individuals, but also in the population and environment. The formulation of future public health measures is one of many areas where multilevel analysis should be used in order to have an appropriate understanding of the effects of area-level factors.

Literature

1. Kaplan, G. A. and J. E. Keil (1993), 'Socioeconomic factors and cardiovascular disease: a review of the literature', *Circulation*, 88, pp. 1973–1998.
2. Kunst, A. E., F. Groenhof, O. Andersen, J. K. Borgan, G. Costa, G. Desplanques, H. Filakti, M. do R. Giraldes, F. Faggiano, S. Harding, C. Junker, P. Martikainen, C. Minder, B. Nolan, F. Pagnanelli, E. Regidor, D. Vagero and T. Valkonen and J. P. Mackenbach (1999), 'Occupational class and ischemic heart disease mortality in the United States and 11 European countries', *American Journal of Public Health*, 89, pp. 47–53.
3. Robinson, W. S. (1950), 'Ecological correlations and the behavior of individuals', *American Sociological Review*, 15, pp. 351–357.
4. Diez-Roux, A. V. (1998), 'Bringing context back into epidemiology: variables and fallacies in multilevel analysis', *American Journal of Public Health*, 88, pp. 216–222.
5. Last, J. M. (2001), *A Dictionary of Epidemiology, 4th ed.*, Oxford: Oxford University Press.
6. Diez-Roux, A. V. (2003), 'The examination of neighborhood effects on health: conceptual and methodological issues related to the presence of multiple levels of organization', in Kawachi Ichirō and Lisa F. Berkman, *Neighborhoods and health*, Oxford: Oxford University Press, pp. 45–64.
7. Blakely, T. A. and A. J. Woodward (2000), 'Ecological effects in multilevel studies', *Journal of Epidemiology and Community Health*, 54, pp. 367–374.
8. Merlo, J., B. Chaix, M. Yang, J. Lynch and L. Rastam (2005), 'A brief conceptual tutorial of multilevel analysis in social epidemiology: linking the statistical concept of clustering to the idea of contextual phenomenon', *Journal of Epidemiology and Community Health*, 59, pp. 443–449.
9. Diez-Roux, A. V. (2002), 'A glossary for multilevel analysis', *Journal of Epidemiology and Community Health*, 56, pp. 588–594.
10. Snijders, T. A. B. and R. J. Bosker (1999), *Multilevel Analysis: An Introduction to Basic and Advanced Multilevel Modelling*, London: Sage.
11. Nishi, N. (1996), 'Metaanarishisu no riron to jissen (The theory and practice of meta-analysis)', *Journal of the Japanese Association for Cerebro-cardiovascular Disease Control*, 30, pp. 192–200.
12. Rasbash, J., F. Steele, W. Browne and B. Prosser (2004), *A User's Guide to MLwiN*, London: Institute of Education, University of London.

13 Martikainen, P., T. M. Kauppinen and T. Valkonen (2003), 'Effects of the characteristics of neighbourhoods and the characteristics of people on cause specific mortality: a register based follow up study of 252,000 men', *Journal of Epidemiology and Community Health*, 57, pp. 210–217.
14 Shibuya, K., H. Hashimoto and E. Yano (2002), 'Individual income, income distribution, and self-rated health in Japan: cross sectional analysis of nationally representative sample', *British Medical Journal*, 324, pp. 16–19.
15 Fukuda, Y., K. Nakamura and T. Takano (2005), 'Accumulation of health risk behaviours is associated with lower socioeconomic status and women's urban residence: a multilevel analysis in Japan', *BMC Public Health*, 5:53 doi: 10.1186/1471–2458/5/53.

11 Social Epidemiology and Individuals, Society and Ethics

Takeo Nakayama

Introduction

In June 2002, the Japanese Ministry of Health, Labour and Welfare (MHLW) and the Japanese Ministry of Education, Culture, Sports, Science and Technology (MEXT) issued the 'Ethical Guidelines for Epidemiological Research' (hereinafter referred to as the Epidemiological Research Guidelines) as a result of collaborative work by epidemiologists, clinical researchers, bioethicists, jurists and, as representatives of the general public, journalists[1].

The Epidemiological Research Guidelines stipulate what procedures should be followed by epidemiological research in order to fulfil its duties as a branch of medicine that conducts research with human subjects. A variety of stakeholders with different interests were involved in the formulation of the guidelines, including those who conduct epidemiological research, those who may be requested to participate in epidemiological research as study subjects, and those who utilise results of epidemiological research. These stakeholders had many discussions and exchanges of views before reaching a consensus[2]. In this process, epidemiologists were asked by people outside the research community the meaning of epidemiology and were faced by the new challenge of explaining to the outside world, in an easy-to-understand manner, the methodology of, and useful results expected from, epidemiological research.

Traditional epidemiology deals mainly with physiological and biochemical indicators, such as lifestyle, blood pressure and serum lipid levels. In contrast, social epidemiology is based on personal information, such as income and education; and this type of information has not been a major concern in conventional epidemiology. While the collection of such information is not physically invasive, it involves potential privacy infringements that cannot be overlooked. This is an issue faced by epidemiological research in general, but is a particularly acute problem in social epidemiological research.

This chapter outlines the history of arguments surrounding the Epidemiological Research Guidelines and protection of personal information in Japan, followed by a summary of issues and points to remember for developing social epidemiological research in an appropriate manner.

The CIOMS Guidelines and the JEA Sub-committee of Ethical Issues

The year 1991 was a significant one for epidemiology, particularly Japanese epidemiology. First, the Japan Epidemiological Association (JEA), which was founded in 1990, held its first annual meeting at the National Cancer Center. This was followed by the release of the 'International Guidelines for Ethical Review of Epidemiological Studies' (hereinafter referred to as the CIOMS Guidelines) by the Council for International Organizations of Medical Sciences (CIOMS)[3, 4].

Background to the formulation of the CIOMS Guidelines can be seen in the preamble section located at: *http://www.cioms.ch/frame_1991_texts_of_guidelines.htm.*

At that time, a serious epidemic of HIV infection in developing countries had triggered a growing global concern about the protection of study participants in vulnerable positions, which had always been an issue in medical studies involving human subjects. The CIOMS Guidelines were particularly significant in that they emphasised the need for the informed consent of study participants, which had not been given full consideration in previous Japanese epidemiological studies. In this regard, the Guidelines seem to have given a shock of some sort to researchers who strived to promote epidemiological studies.

In response to the CIOMS Guidelines, during the first half of the 1990s Japan saw several early attempts to measure the degree of compliance with informed consent requirements in epidemiological studies[5]. The Japan Collaborative Cohort Study for the Evaluation of Cancer Risk (JACC Study)[6] was started in 1988 by the Special Cancer Research Organization, which was sponsored by the Grant-in-Aid for Scientific Research Program of the Japanese Ministry of Education, Science, Sports and Culture (MESC, the predecessor of MEXT). Within this study, a questionnaire survey of researchers was conducted in 1993 to measure the degree of compliance with informed consent requirements in requests to participants in various field studies. The survey was carried out by the Japan Epidemiological Association's (Sub-)Committee of Ethical Issues, and the results were reported at the 1996 International Scientific Meeting of the International Epidemiological Association held in Nagoya[7, 8]. The main findings included: (1) in almost all cohorts, informed consent was obtained for the questionnaire survey on health, but in different manners in different cohorts; (2) in 28 of the 34 cohorts, informed consent was obtained for submission of blood samples for storage; and (3) the researchers chose not to use samples for which informed consent had not been obtained.

As described above, at that time informed consent was the focus of epidemiologists' attention in terms of research ethics. It seems that scarcely any attention was paid to the protection of personal information, and this soon became an issue. It also seems that there was no clear pressure from outside the epidemiological research community to establish principles of research ethics. Most of the efforts made at that time are likely to have been voluntary ones made by researchers inspired by the CIOMS Guidelines.

Early efforts towards research ethics guidelines (1997–2000)

Background

In the latter half of the 1990s, younger researchers in the JEA played a key role in promoting active discussions on informed consent issues and research ethics[9]. In April 1998, the Study on the Development of Ethics Guidelines for Informed Consent in Epidemiologic Research was set up as a scientific research project sponsored by the Japanese Ministry of Health and Welfare (MHW, predecessor of the MHLW). This Study was led by Akiko Tamakoshi, who served as chief researcher for the project. The project team is hereinafter referred to as the Tamakoshi Team. With this, the movement towards the development of ethical guidelines swung into full gear. The Tamakoshi Team consisted mainly of young and mid-level epidemiologists of the JEA. They were joined by some young researchers in bioethics and law. Their main topic of discussion was informed consent issues in cohort studies and other observational studies. This writer was one of the epidemiologists who participated in the Tamakoshi Team.

It was at that time when the movement towards the legislation of a personal information protection law rapidly became active.

In July 1999, the Personal Information Protection Investigative Subcommittee was established in the Advanced Information and Telecommunications Society Promotion Headquarters headed by the Prime Minister. In November of the same year, the Subcommittee issued an interim report, 'The modality of a personal information protection system in Japan' (in Japanese, *'Wagakuni niokeru kojin jōhō hogo shisutemu no arikata nitsuite'*), which pointed out the necessity for the enactment of a basic law for the protection of personal information.

The movement towards the legislation of a personal information protection law in Japan dates back to 1980, when the OECD (Organization for Economic Cooperation and Development) adopted the Recommendation of the Council concerning Guidelines Governing the Protection of Privacy and Transborder Flows of Personal Data (the OECD's 8 Principles). In 1995 the EU adopted 'Directive 95/46/EC on the protection of individuals with regard to the processing of personal data and on the free movement of such data', which meant that EU member states had to legislate for a personal information protection system by 1998, and that the transfer of personal information to a non-EU country would be permitted only if the country had taken satisfactory protection measures. In order to maintain exchanges with the EU member states, Japan had an increased necessity to legislate a personal information protection system. The MHW and some epidemiologists pointed out that the aforementioned interim report was under the direct influence of the OECD's 8 Principles, as seen in the 'principle of consent' (which derived from the 'individual participation principle') applicable to the collection of personal information, and warned that direct application of the report might pose substantial restrictions on epidemiological studies which provide a basis for public health in areas such as disease registration and cohort studies[10, 11].

The impact of personal information protection on public health

Of all public health issues, cancer registration is most notably affected by the issue of personal information protection. To obtain least-biased information on cancer incidence and prognosis, it is desirable, in terms of policy, to establish a cancer registration system completely on a survey basis. However, not all patients are notified of their diagnosis. For this reason, application of the 'principle of consent' to the collection of personal information would greatly shake the foundation of a cancer registration system.

We can learn a lesson from the breakdown of the cancer registration system in Hamburg (in the former West Germany) in 1980[10]. In 1977 in Hamburg, the Act for the Prevention of Misuse of Personal Data in Data Processing, which was similar to the OECD's 8 Principles, was enacted. This Act applied the principle of consent to the reporting of patient information. This resulted in a rapid decrease in the number of reports, from about 10,000 reports per year to only two in 1980–1981, leading to a virtual breakdown of the system. Later, in 1986, the Chernobyl nuclear disaster occurred in the former Soviet Union, increasing the need for information on cancer incidence. However, there was no longer a system that could scientifically assess potential exposure and its effect on cancer incidence at the population level[11].

In 1979 in the USA, Professor Leon Gordis of the Johns Hopkins University testified at a hearing before the Government Information and Individual Rights Subcommittee of the US Congress in support of epidemiological research, its methodology and its significance for society[12]. Gordis took as an example a case-control study that demonstrated the toxicity of DES (diethyl stilbestrol)[13], which was later classified as a Class I carcinogenic by the International Agency for Research on Cancer (IARC). Gordis warned that requiring the patients' consent in accessing past medical records might hinder prompt discovery of health risks.

Thus, Western countries were about two decades ahead of Japan in being concerned that the issue of personal information protection would have a serious impact on epidemiology. Under the circumstances, Japanese epidemiologists and the MHW aimed at having epidemiological studies exempted from the application of some of the principles of personal information protection, without resisting the overall trend towards personal information protection. A similar policy was adopted for public health activities and medical research as in EU directives and the Standards for Privacy of Individually Identifiable Health Information issued by the US Department of Health and Human Services in 1999.

Social accountability and background to research ethics guidelines

In the latter half of 1999, genetic analysis that had been conducted in epidemiological studies became an issue in Japan after media coverage of cases of genetic research without the subjects' consent. A leading national newspaper ran on their front page a series of reports on several cases of un-consented genetic analysis of blood samples collected for mass screening[14-16]. It can be inferred that these

Table 11.1: Recommendations for the role of epidemiology in the 21st century

1. In compliance with personal information protection law and other related laws, regulations and guidelines, and
2. in close cooperation with society, epidemiology for the 21st century should
3. ensure appropriate utilisation of information,
4. produce results that meet the trust and expectation of society,
5. while fulfilling accountability as epidemiologists, and
6. feed the results back into society in a visible manner.

Source: *Ekigaku kenkyū no gyōsei-teki sokumen kara no hyōka ni kansuru kenkyū*, special research sponsored by the Japanese Ministry of Health and Welfare, 1999.

events and the press coverage gave a negative first impression of epidemiology to people who had been unaware of its existence.

Under the circumstances, this author took charge of the 'Study on Assessment of Epidemiologic Research in terms of Contributions to Health Policy', which was initiated hastily in January 2000 as a special research program sponsored by the MHW. The Study retrospectively reviewed the results of epidemiological studies and their application to national policy from the viewpoint of accountability to society[17]. The Study also outlined 'etiologic epidemiology' and 'policy epidemiology' proposed by the Canadian epidemiologist Robert Spasoff[18]. Based on Spasoff's theory, we discussed the possibility of a new epidemiology which would focus on contributing to policy-making, as opposed to traditional epidemiology which aimed at elucidation of the causes of diseases. The discussion resulted in six recommendations for the future role of epidemiology (Table 11.1).

In March 2000, the Committee for Advanced Medical Technology Assessment of the Health Sciences Council established an *ad hoc* committee on privacy protection in scientific studies using epidemiologic methodology. In addition, the JEA posted a statement on its website explaining to the general public the relationship between epidemiology and personal information, and seeking the exemption of personal information in epidemiological studies from a basic law on personal information protection, and related laws and regulations[19]. In April the same year, the MHW Tamakoshi Team published *Ekigaku kenkyū ni okeru infōmudo konsento ni kansuru gaidorain ver. 1.0* ('Guidelines on informed consent in epidemiological studies, ver. 1.0'), as the product of the team's two-year activities[20]. In the formulation of their Guidelines, the Tamakoshi Team first emphasised the process of informed consent which respected the CIOMS Guidelines while taking Japan's actual situation into account. However, their final work took into consideration the aspect of personal information protection as well, as this issue rapidly gained significance during the latter half of the Guidelines drafting process. Subsequently, the MHW set up the Project Team for the Study of Ethical Ramifications and Personal Data Protection in Research and Programs Using Epidemiologic Methods (hereinafter referred to as the 'Maruyama Team' named after the chief researcher, Eiji Maruyama, a professor at Kobe University). While the Tamakoshi Team focused on the issue of informed consent in observational studies, the Maruyama Team discussed ethical issues in epidemiological methods in general, including intervention studies. In addition, while the Tamakoshi Team was characterised by its emphasis on the autonomy of researchers, the Maruyama Team focused on the formulation of guidelines based on the spirit of the Personal Information Protection Bill, in order to deal with the issue of personal information protection.

In October 2000, the Japanese government's Personal Information Protection Legislation Expert Committee issued an outline of the proposed Personal Information Protection Bill. The outline consisted of five basic principles applicable to both the official and private sectors, and the obligations to be imposed on businesses. In response, in March 2001, the Science Council of Japan – 7th Division (Medicine, Dentistry and Pharmaceutical Science) released a statement titled 'The Modality of Legislation Concerning the Protection of Personal Information in Medical Research'. The statement warned that imposing the obligations of 'personal information handling businesses' on medical research institutions and individual researchers would have a serious impact on the development of medical research, and urged that medical research be exempted from the application of the basic principles and the obligations to be imposed on personal information handling businesses[21]. Similar statements were issued by other organisations, including the Japanese Society of Public Health, the Japan Society for Occupational Health[22], and the Japanese Association of Directors of Departments of Hygiene and Public Health at Medical Schools.

As mentioned above, during those few years, the JEA, MHW and MESC worked on reconfirming the social significance of epidemiology, and on issuing statements to the outside world, amid the pincer attack (so to speak) from the overall trend towards legislation for a personal information protection law (which arose because of overseas demands), and media coverage reporting unconsented analysis of samples in epidemiological studies. This was an important period in which epidemiologists were asked by people outside the research community about the meaning of epidemiology, and hence, started to work on the question.

The Maruyama Team and the IMJC: establishing ethical guidelines

Creation of the MEXT/MHLW Joint Committee

In March 2001, the MHLW, MEXT and Ministry of Economy, Trade and Industry (METI) issued the Ethical Guidelines for Analytical Research on Human Genome/Genes. Just previously, in April 2000, the Maruyama Team, after more than ten meetings, issued the Guidelines for Personal Information Protection and Bioethical Issues in Epidemiologic Research (the Maruyama Team Guidelines)[23]. Initially, the Maruyama Team Guidelines were meant to be applied widely to studies sponsored by the MHLW. However, the Maruyama Team Guidelines did not eventually come into effect due to demands from clinical researchers for revision of the requirement that the use of existing documents, including medical records maintained at their own medical centres, undergo ethical review. The Maruyama Team Guidelines also established a policy that ethical guidelines for epidemiology and for clinical studies should be discussed separately.

Based on the results of work done by the Maruyama Team, in May 2001 the MHLW established another *ad hoc* Committee on the Implementation of Research Using Epidemiologic Methods, which was under the jurisdiction of the Science and Technology Panel of the MHLW Health Sciences Council (hereinafter referred to as the MHLW Committee). At the instigation of MEXT in March 2001, the Association of Japanese Medical Colleges set up a subcommittee for the formulation of its own ethical guidelines. This subcommittee was taken over by the Subcommittee on Studies Using Epidemiological Methods, which was established in the Bioethics and Biosafety Commission of the Council for Science and Technology. After its first discussion, the new subcommittee decided on a policy to hold joint discussions with the MHLW Committee. The joint committee was called the Expert Committee on Appropriate Promotion of Studies Using Epidemiological Methods (hereinafter referred to as the Inter-

Ministry Joint Committee, or IMJC). The IMJC played the final role in formulating ethical guidelines for epidemiology[24, 25].

The office of the IMJC was served by representatives from both ministries and the Committee consisted of representatives from the following fields: epidemiology (3 representatives), clinical medicine (8), nursing science (1), law (5) and mass media (2). After discussion and deliberation, the members agreed on the necessity for guidelines that would reflect the increased public awareness of the right of privacy and personal information protection. The IMJC decided to name the proposed guidelines the 'Ethical Guidelines for Epidemiological Research'.

The scope of their application was determined as follows: 'These guidelines shall apply to all epidemiological studies aiming to elucidate the etiology and pathology of, and to establish prevention and treatment methods for, human diseases, and must be complied with by all parties involved in these studies'. An epidemiological study could be exempted from the Guidelines in the following cases:

1. a survey conducted in accordance with the provisions of any law;
2. a study conducted in accordance with the Ethical Guidelines for Analytical Research on Human Genome/Genes (Notification No.1 of the MHLW, MEXT and METI of 2004);
3. a study based solely on de-identified information (i.e. information de-linked from the identity of the subjects); or
4. an intervention study involving surgery, medication or other medical treatment.

An outline of the Ethical Guidelines for Epidemiological Research

As a result of IMJC discussions, the following provisions were included in the Guidelines. In principle, the subjects' informed consent must be obtained in each epidemiological study. This requirement may be relaxed or exempted subject to certain conditions. When any relaxation or exemption applies, the researchers must, depending on the research methods, make written records of informed consent and relevant information available to the public, and provide the subjects with opportunities to refuse participation in the study. In observational studies using existing samples, researchers are not always required to obtain informed consent and, if not, must make information on the conduct of the study available to the public.

Regarding the Personal Information Protection Bill, the Guidelines provided that colleges, universities and research institutions would be exempted from the proposed obligations to be imposed on businesses, and that the Guidelines should be regarded as one of the 'guidelines established by the government in order to support colleges, universities and other academic research institutions to take effective measures for personal information protection', as set out in Article 13 of the Bill. 'De-identification' was defined as 'to replace all or part of the personal identification information of a subject's personal information with a code or number that is not associated with the subject'. However, no provisions were included in the Guidelines as to who should be responsible for de-identification or who should be responsible for personal information protection. The Guidelines provided that they should not apply to any investigation of medical records for the primary purpose of discussing therapeutic measures for specific or non-specific patients. A cancer registration project was defined as 'a health project which collects and organises data from medical institutions', and was exempted. However, it was stipulated that an epidemiological study which analyses data from a cancer registration project to test a hypothesis would be subject to the Guidelines.

Concerning the ethical review boards (ERBs), the Two Ministry Joint Committee discussed review procedures, the composition of board members, problems with existing ERBs, and an appropriate review process for multi-centre studies. The final provisions included in the Guidelines were that the researchers should submit their research project to the head of their institution, who should file an application for ethical review with the relevant ERB, and that an ERB should consist of experts in Medicine, Humanities and Social Science, representatives of the general public and external members, and should include both male and female members. The head of each research institution was obligated to establish an ERB, but it was provided in the operational regulations that if the establishment of an ERB by the centres is impracticable in a multi-centre study, ethical review may be requested of an ERB jointly created by the centres involved in the study.

After the activities described above, the Ethical Guidelines for Epidemiological Research were completed in June 2002. Strict application of the Epidemiological Research Guidelines is required for epidemiological studies sponsored by public funds, including

Table 11.2: Ethical declaration on the conduct of epidemiological research

All epidemiological research must:
1. aim at pursuing the truth;
2. respect the subjects' human rights;
3. use the most appropriate methods to accomplish its objectives;
4. not violate social norms; and
5. always be open to society.

Source: The Japan Epidemiological Association's website.

MEXT or MHLW research projects. However, the scope of application is not limited to these publicly funded studies. The Guidelines state that 'all parties involved in epidemiological studies are requested to engage in their studies in compliance with these guidelines, in order that epidemiological research may gain understanding and trust from, and make further contributions to, society'.

Since creating the Epidemiological Research Guidelines

In response to the completion of the Epidemiological Research Guidelines, Japanese colleges, universities and research institutions promptly proceeded with the development of ethics review systems. In October 2002, the JEA announced the Ethical Guidelines for the Conduct of Epidemiological Research, which had been formulated in a manner consistent with the Epidemiological Research Guidelines. The JEA Guidelines declared that an ERB would be established in the JEA (Table 11.2). This enabled researchers from organisations without an ethics review system to go through such a review, subject to their membership with the JEA.

During the 155th session of the Japanese Diet in 2002, the Bill on the Protection of Personal Information, or the Personal Information Protection Basic Bill, was shelved and abandoned. This was partly due to objections from the media, which had concerns about the potential impact on their freedom of news gathering. Subsequently, the Bill was amended by replacing all five 'basic principles', including 'restrictions depending on the purpose of use' and 'proper collection', with the 'basic philosophy' that the proper handling of personal information must be pursued. The amended bill was resubmitted to the Diet during its 156th session in March 2003 and became law in May as the Act on the Protection of Personal Information. In the Act, academic research, together with press activities, writing, religious and political activities are exempted from the obligations imposed on 'personal information handling businesses'. Instead, the Act provides that each academic research program has an obligation to strive to take necessary measures independently and to make details of such measures available to the public. For the Japanese epidemiological community, the establishment of its Epidemiological Research Guidelines constituted a thorough effort to fulfil this obligation. The Epidemiological Research Guidelines were revised in December 2004, in order to ensure consistency with the Personal Information Protection Act, which was due for enforcement in April 2005.

Needless to say, not only epidemiology but all other fields of medicine were required to establish their own code of conduct for research. In former times, there were no clear norms or standards other than the Declaration of Helsinki as the basic principles, the Japanese Pharmaceutical Affairs Law regulating clinical studies, and new ordinances and regulations relating to GCP (Good Clinical Practice) (*http://www.mhlw.go.jp/shingi/2005/03/dl/s0329-13l.pdf*). The Epidemiological Research Guidelines and the Ethical Guidelines for Clinical Studies (the latter being established soon after the establishment of the Epidemiological Research Guidelines) helped to establish the scope of, and organise methods for, medical research involving human subjects, not only within the research community, but also in a manner visible to the outside world. While some activities, such as the aforementioned cancer registration programs or medical review studies based on field clinical activities, are difficult to be classified into any one category, the construction of the above framework seems to be a sign of the maturity of medical research in that it enhances the transparency and accountability of medical research to society. The traditional mission of epidemiological research has been to find out the causes of diseases. In the future, additional tasks of epidemiological research, such as establishing its social position and communicating with parties that should be directly benefiting from the research (policymakers and the general public), are likely to become more significant[26].

Ethical issues in social epidemiology research

Use of public statistics

As described above, issues concerning the ethical requirements (mainly for personal information protection) of epidemiological research in general are becoming clearer. Some issues have been settled to a certain extent, while others require further discussion. The Act on the Protection of Personal Information and the Epidemiological Research Guidelines share the same definition of personal information: 'information on a living individual which allows identification of the individual from the name, date of birth and/or any other data included in it (including information which can readily be linked with other information and which allows identification of a specific individual through such linkage)'. In this section, I would like to review these issues from the viewpoint of social epidemiology which aims at the elucidation of the effects of socioeconomic factors on health.

Epidemiological studies, including social epidemiological studies, can be broadly categorised into two. First, there are ecological studies, which formulate epidemiological hypotheses based on the correlation between or among the respective representative values of two or more populations (e.g. the correlation between the average salt intake and the proportion of people with high blood pressure or the average blood pressure value, and the correlation between the amount of fish consumption and the incidence of depression). Secondly, there are analytical epidemiological studies (i.e. cohort studies and case-control studies) which test epidemiological hypotheses by linking exposure information and prognosis information at the individual level. In an ecological study which analyses population-level data using existing public statistics, individuals cannot be identified. Thus, information used in this type of study does not fall under the definition of personal information. This type of study is not subject to ethical review, as it falls under Item 3 of the aforementioned exemptions listed in the Epidemiological Research Guidelines, that is, 'a study based solely on de-identified information, i.e. information de-linked from the identity of the subjects'. However, activities to systematically collect this type of information in preparatory stages of a study are significantly affected by the Personal Information Protection Act and the increased awareness of privacy in society. Examples of this effect include the declining rates of cooperation and/or participation in the National Census, the Comprehensive Survey of Living Conditions of the People on Health and Welfare, and the National Nutrition Survey. These surveys, including the National Census, which is a component of 'designated statistics' (i.e. statistics generated by the national and local governments, those designated by the Minister of Public Management, Home Affairs, Posts and

Telecommunications as necessary for the determination of basic national policy), fall under Item 1 of the exemptions listed in the Epidemiological Research Guidelines: 'a survey conducted in accordance with the provisions of any law'. The appropriate conduct of these surveys and the appropriate use of information collected from these surveys for research are secured by laws and ethical guidelines. However, the social awareness of privacy has been making the smooth conduct of these statistical surveys difficult. It can pose a threat not only to social epidemiological and biomedical research but also to policymaking by the national and local governments. This is an issue requiring public discussion.

Linking personal information

Since analytical epidemiology involves linking exposure information and outcome (or prognosis) information at an individual level, activities involved in analytical epidemiological studies are broadly categorised into two types which are associated with the respective types of information. In general, exposure information is collected directly from individual subjects using questionnaires. In contrast, outcome information is usually collected by accessing such sources as medical records, itemized statements of medical expenses, and death certificates, due to the nature of this type of information pertaining to diseases and death. An individual's exposure information can only be collected with their consent. Conversely, once the subject's consent is duly obtained, researchers are free to collect and use exposure information in their study. The Epidemiological Research Guidelines detail different forms of informed consent required for different research methods and objectives. The subject matters of social epidemiological studies include people's economic, educational and working status, and quite a few subjects refuse to answer questions on these matters as they do not want to disclose such information to others. In Japan as well as other countries, epidemiological studies focusing on the elucidation of the effects of social factors on health have collected information on exposure factors. However, this type of information has been collected only in a very limited number of cases in epidemiological studies focusing on lifestyles and molecular epidemiological studies emphasising gene polymorphism.

Some say the collection of private information in epidemiological studies is ethically wrong in itself, but I think this is an extreme argument. Examples of the definitions of privacy include: '(1)

personal affairs, private life, and secrets; and (2) the legal right to protect secrets and honour in one's private life from third parties'; and a 'state of not being disturbed by any other person and not being paid attention by the public'. Epidemiological studies are based on subjects' personal information which is, in a sense, private information that they may not want others to know. Privacy information may include not only income and education but also obesity level, smoking or drinking history, and exercise behaviour. Making all these items of information inaccessible because of privacy would make all fields of medical research unfeasible, including epidemiological research, which aims at solving these medical problems. In addition, there are cases where researchers need to access highly private information in order to identify and delineate the actual situation of issues which have been concealed from the eyes of community members but have actually troubled many people. For instance, some two decades ago, 'dementia (cognitive disorder) in elderly people' and 'burdens on caregivers' were still generally concealed in society. These were regarded as problems for individual families and households, and constituted private information that they wanted to conceal from others. However, if their situations had remained invisible, no social measures could ever have been taken. After the 1980s, epidemiological studies were conducted widely in Japan by the national, prefectural and municipal governments, many of which were conducted as local government-led administrative investigations without the involvement of researchers. These studies helped to distribute knowledge and information widely on the social impact of elderly dementia and the burdens of caregivers. This later had an impact on the medical programs and promoted the establishment of the nursing care insurance system. In the future, a similar process may be followed for such issues as domestic violence and child abuse. Promotion of social awareness of these issues and some counter-measures will require a solid foundation of further development of descriptive and analytical epidemiology.

    Needless to say, when researchers access any private information, it is imperative that they provide the subjects with sufficient explanation of the necessity of such access for public health purposes, and give sufficient consideration to the collection and management of such information, and to maintain its confidentiality. In addition, it is desirable that any questionnaires include a statement to the effect that the subject is requested to answer the questions on a totally voluntary basis and may choose not to answer any or all of the questions at his/her discretion (but that the subject is encouraged to understand the aim of the survey and to answer as many questions as possible). This is in sharp contrast to questionnaires used only a decade ago which demanded the subject answer all questions. However, the current questionnaires increase the risk of a strong bias. If a collected questionnaire includes unanswered questions, researchers cannot tell whether the subject chose not to answer or simply forgot to answer the questions. If the latter situation is the case, they may have to ask the subject the same questions again to find out his/her answers. As a measure to deal with this kind of situation, a questionnaire could include an instruction to mark an X in the answer column if the subject intentionally chooses not to answer. In any case, in the field of social epidemiology, further consideration and discussion is desirable concerning appropriate measures for collecting information for different study objectives and from study subjects in different situations.

The subjects of social epidemiological studies include people's economic, educational and working status. In current circumstances, where personal information protection is trumpeted, access to information on these matters may generate additional ethical issues further along in the process, from data collection to giving feedback to the community. Since the enforcement of the Personal Information Protection Act in April 2005, several problems have been pointed out in which excessive adjustments to the Act have caused friction in various parts of our social lives[27]. This is associated with concern about the potential effects on requisite research activities. Researchers in each field of study are requested to take measures as soon as a new issue arises or in some cases, take preliminary measures beforehand. Researchers in social epidemiology are requested to ask themselves what findings they can feed back into the community or what contributions they can make to the community through the development of social epidemiological research, and to answer these questions for the study subjects and the community at large in an easy-to-understand manner.

In future, researchers in epidemiology will be further required to make continuous efforts to reconsider the significance of epidemiology, and to convey to the community the contents and meanings of their research activities, based on the Epidemiology Research Guidelines, and through their activities, to formulate, modify and implement these Guidelines.

Acknowledgements

I am grateful to Professor Masahiro Takaishi, Professor Yutaka Inaba, Dr. Kiyotaka Segami, Professor Eiji Maruyama and Dr. Akiko Tamakoshi for their valuable advice on my paper published in the *Journal of Epidemiology*, on which this chapter is based. I would also like to thank Ms Michi Sakai and Mr Brian Slingsby for their great cooperation in organising and studying the related documents.

Literature

1. The Japanese Ministry of Health, Labour and Welfare and the Japanese Ministry of Education, Culture, Sports, Science and Technology (2002), 'Ekigaku kenkyū ni kansuru rinri shishin (Ethical Guidelines for Epidemiological Research)'.
2. Nakayama, T., M. Sakai and B. T. Slingsby (2005), 'Japan's ethical guidelines for epidemiologic research: a history of their development', *Journal of Epidemiology*, 15 (4), pp. 107-112.
3. CIOMS (The Council for International Organizations of Medical Sciences) (1991), International Guidelines for Ethical Review of Epidemiologic Studies. Geneva.
4. CIOMS (1991), International Guidelines for Ethical Review of Epidemiologic Studies, (Translated by Tadahiro Mitsuishi, 1992: *Rinshō Hyōka*, Clinical Evaluation), 20 (3), pp. 563–578).
5. Nakayama, T., K. Mutō, N. Yoshiike and T. Yokoyama (1999), 'Awareness and motivation of Japanese donors of blood for research', *American Journal of Public Health*, 89, pp. 1433–1434.
6. Ohno, Y., A. Tamakoshi and the JACC Study Group (2001), 'Japan collaborative cohort study for evaluation of cancer risk sponsored by the Monbusho (JACC study)', *Journal of Epidemiology*, 11 (4), pp. 144–150.
7. Subcommittee of Ethical Issues (1996), 'What ethical issues are Japanese epidemiologists facing?: Results of a questionnaire study for members of the Monbusho Research Committee on evaluation of risk factors for cancer by large-scale cohort study', *Journal of Epidemiology*, 6, (3 Suppl), pp. S141–146.
8. Inaba, Y. (1996), 'Recent topics in Japan', *Journal of Epidemiology*, 6 (3 Suppl), pp. S137–139.
9. Kobashi, G., T. Hoshuyama, H. Sugimori, I. Oki, T. Kadowaki, H. Kanda, T. Otani, M. Iwasaki, M. Naito and S. Takao (2004), 'What expectations do young Japanese epidemiologists have for the future of epidemiology? A questionnaire survey of members of the young epidemiologists society for discussing the future of epidemiology', *Journal of Epidemiology*, 14 (2), pp. 69–71.
10. Segami, K., T. Satō, A. Ichinose and T. Ōtake (2000), 'Kōshūeisei to kojin jōhō hogo no enkaku to kongo no arikata (The history and future of public health and personal information protection)', *Kōshū Eisei* (The Journal of Public Health Practice), 64 (8), pp. 532–540.

11 Mizushima, S. (2000), 'Kojin jōhō to dēta no rikatsuyō ni kansuru kokusaiteki dōkō (International trends in the use of personal information and data)', *Kōshū Eisei* (The Journal of Public Health Practice), 64, pp. 548–556.
12 Gordis, L. and E. Gold (1980), 'Privacy, confidentiality, and the use of medical records in research', *Science*, 207 (4427), pp. 153–156.
13 Herbst, A. L., H. Ulfelder and D. C. Poskanzer (1971), 'Adenocarcinoma of the vagina: Association of maternal stilbestrol therapy with tumor appearance in young women', *New England Journal of Medicine*, 284 (15), pp. 878–881.
14 *Asahi Shimbun* (26 October 1999), 'Jūmin no idenshi mudan kaiseki: kōketsuatsu no kenkyū ni kenshin no saiketsu tsukau (Unconsented gene analysis of residents: blood samples from mass screening used in hypertension study)'.
15 *Mainichi Shimbun* (3 February 2000), 'Kokuritsu junkankibyō sentā ga idenshi 5000 nin bun wo mudan kaiseki (National Cardiovascular Center analyzed genes of 5000 patients without consent'.
16 *Kyōdō News* (8 March 2000), Karute wo mudan de etsuran: junkanki shikkan no ekigaku chōsa (Unconsented access to medical records: epidemiological survey of cardiovascular disease).
17 1999-nendo Kōseikagaku Tokubetsu Kenkyū (MHLW Special Research Program for FY 1999) (chief researcher, Takeo Nakayama) (1999), 'Gyōseiteki sokumen kara mita ekigaku kenkyū no hyōka ni kansuru kenkyū (A Study on Assessment of Epidemiologic Research in terms of Contributions to Health Policy)'.
18 Spasoff, R. (1999), *Epidemiologic Methods for Health Policy*, Oxford: Oxford University Press, (Translation edited by T. Uehata, translated by S. Mizushima, Y. Michizuki, T. Nakayama et al. 2003, Tokyo: Igaku Shoin).
19 Japan Epidemiological Association (2000), 'Kojin jōhō hogo ni kanren suru hō seibi ni kansuru seimei (A statement on the development of legal systems relating to personal information protection)', *http://www.soc.nii.ac.jp/jea/main/seimei/html*, accessed 27 October 2005.
20 Ekigaku Kenkyū ni okeru Infōmudo Konsento ni kansuru Kenkyū to Rinri Gaidorain Sakutei Kenkyūhan (A Study on the Development of Ethics Guidelines for Informed Consent in Epidemiologic Research) (2000), *Ekigaku kenkyū ni okeru infōmudo konsento ni kansuru gaidorain ver. 1.0* (Guidelines on Informed Consent in Epidemiological Studies, ver. 1.0), Tokyo: Nihon Iji Shinpō Sha.
21 The Science Council of Japan the 7th Division (2001), 'Igaku kenkyū kara mita kojin jōhō no hogo ni kansuru hōsei no arikata ni tsuite (Legislation on the protection of personal information from the viewpoint of medical research)', *http://www.scj.go.jp/kennkyuusyasaronnr/18pdf/1865.pdf*, accessed 27 October 2005.
22 Japan Society for Occupational Health (2000), Kojin jōhō hogo kihon hō seitei ni tsuite no yōbōsho (Requests regarding the proposed enactment of a personal information protection basic act), *http://www.sanei.or.jp/topics/topicdocument.html*, accessed 27 October 2005.
23 Ekigakuteki Shuhō wo Mochiita Kenkyū tō ni okeru Seimei Rinri Mondai oyobi Kojin Jōhō Hogo no Arikata ni Kansuru Chōsa Kenkyūhan (Project

Team for Bioethics and Personal Information Protection Issues in Studies Using Epidemiological Methods) (2001), Ekigaku no kenkyū tō ni okeru seimei rinri mondai oyobi kojin jōhō hogo no arikata ni kansuru shishin (an) (Guidelines on bioethics and personal information protection issues in epidemiological and other studies – draft), 10 April 2001 version.

24 Kenkyū Rinri ni Kansuru Shōiinkai (Subcommittee on Research Ethics of the Association of Japanese Medical Colleges (2003), 'Ekigaku kenkyū tō ni kansuru gaidorain shian (Draft guidelines on epidemiological research)', *Kōshū Eisei Kenyū* (Journal of National Institute of Public Health), 52 (3), pp. 224-227.

25 Inaba, Y. (2003), 'Ekigaku kenkyū ni kansuru rinri shishin: sakusei no keii (Ethical Guidelines for Epidemiological Research: the background of formulation)', *Kōshū Eisei Kenyū* (Journal of National Institute of Public Health), 52 (3), pp. 183–186.

26 Naitō, M., T. Nakayama, T. Ojima, G. Kobashi, K. Muto, M. Washio, S. Ishikawa, E. Maruyama, M. Sakai, K. Sato, H. Sugimori, M. Suzuki, F. Takahashi, Z. Yamagata and A. Tamakoshi (2004), 'Creating a brochure to promote understanding of epidemiological research', *Journal of Epidemiology*, 14 (5), pp. 174–176.

26 *Yomiuri Shimbun* (20 August 2005), 'Kojin jōhō hogo, kajō han'nō!? aitsugu (A succession of overreactions(!?) to personal information protection act'.

Appendix

Table A.1: List of major events in and outside Japan relating to the establishment of the Japanese Ethical Guidelines for Epidemiological Research

1947	The Nuremberg Code emphasizes the protection of human research subjects out of regret for the Nazis' inhuman experimentation on people.
1954	Willowbrook Experiment (mentally disabled children were intentionally infected with hepatitis virus at a state-supported institution for mentally retarded children in New York).
1963	The Jewish Chronic Disease Hospital Case (an experiment in which live cancer cells were injected into terminally ill patients at the Jewish Chronic Disease Hospital of Brooklyn, New York).
1964	The World Medical Association's Declaration of Helsinki emphasises the importance of informed consent.
Late 1960s	The issue of personal information protection is raised out of concern for management of electronic personal information, mainly in Germany, Sweden and the Netherlands.
1972	Tuskegee Syphilis Experiment occurs in the US state of Alabama. (An article titled 'Syphilis Victims in the U.S. Study Went Untreated for 40 Years' ran on the front page of the New York Times).
Apr. 1979	Prof. Gordis of Johns Hopkins University testifies about the methodology and significance of epidemiology before the US Congress Subcommittee on Government Information And Individual Rights.
	Office of the Secretary of the US Department of Health, Education and Welfare issues the Ethical Principles and Guidelines for the Protection of Human Subjects of Research (Belmont Report) based on investigation of the Tuskegee Syphilis Experiment.
Sep. 1980	OECD Europe adopts the OECD Recommendation Concerning, and Guidelines Governing, the Protection of Privacy and Transborder Flows of Personal Data.
1982	CIOMS issues the International Ethical Guidelines for Biomedical Research Involving Human Subjects.
1989	'Ethical Issues in Preventive Medicine' study project is sponsored by the Japanese Ministry of Education, Science, Sports and Culture (MESC) (chief researcher, Shun'ichi Yamamoto).

Table A.1: continued

1990	The Japan Epidemiological Association (JEA) is founded.
	The Japanese Ministry of Labour sets up a study on the prevention of work-related diseases, including cardiovascular disease.
Jan. 1991	The JEA holds its 1st annual meeting (at the National Cancer Center, Tokyo).
1991	CIOMS issues the International Guidelines for Ethical Review of Epidemiological Studies.
	Prof. Guyatt (Canada) publishes 'Evidence-based Medicine' in ACP (American College of Physicians) Journal Club.
1993	A survey is conducted with the purpose of evaluating the process of informed consent in the large-scale study 'The Collaborative Cohort Study for Evaluation of Cancer Risk' (the predecessor of the JACC Study).
	CIOMS revises the International Ethical Guidelines for Biomedical Research Involving Human Subjects.
Nov. 1995	EU adopts 'Directive 95/46/EC on the protection of individuals with regard to the processing of personal data and on the free movement of such data'.
Jan. 1996	The young members of the JEA held the first research meeting entitled 'Informed consent in epidemiological studies' at the sixth JEA conference in Nagoya.
Aug. 1996	The International Scientific Meeting of the International Epidemiological Association (IEA) is held in Nagoya, Japan. Results of the 1993 survey are presented.
Jan. 1997	At the 7th JEA annual meeting (in Tokyo), the second young researchers' study meeting is held under the theme 'Informed Consent in Epidemiological Studies'.
Jan. 1998	The 2nd Asia-Pacific Conference of IEA and the 8th annual meeting of JEA are both held in Tokyo. The third young researchers' study meeting is held under the theme 'Informed Consent in Epidemiological Studies'.
Apr. 1998	The 'Development of Ethics Guidelines for Informed Consent in Epidemiologic Research' is set up as a research project sponsored by MHW.
Aug. 1998	The amended Basic Resident Registration Law is passed by the Japanese coalition government consisting of the Liberal Democratic Party, the Liberal Party and the New Kōmeitō Party.
May 1999	The Health Sciences Council issues the statement titiled 'The MHW future modality towards the 21st Century'.
Jun. 1999	The Advanced Information and Telecommunications Society Promotion Headquarters establishes the Personal Information Protection Investigative Subcommittee (chaired by Masao Horibe, a professor at Chūō University).

Table A.1: continued

Nov. 1999	The above subcommittee issues the interim report.
	The Asahi Shimbun runs an article titled 'Genetic analysis of citizen DNA without permission: Use of blood taken at health checkups for research on high blood pressure'. This is followed by many other reports by Japanese national newspapers of unconsented gene analysis cases in epidemiological studies.
Dec. 1999	The then Prime Minister Keizō Obuchi set up the Millenium Project focusing on information technology, aging and the environment.
Jan. 2000	The JEA establishes the *ad hoc* Committee on Ethical Issues (chaired by Yutaka Inaba).
	The 'Study on assessment of epidemiologic research in terms of contributions to health policy' is set up as a research project sponsored by MHW.
Mar. 2000	National Cancer Center Symposium, public symposium (e.g. personal information protection in epidemiologic research such as cancer registries) is held.
	The Health Sciences Council Committee for Advanced Medical Technology Assessment establishes the *ad hoc* Committee on Privacy Protection in Research Using Epidemiologic Methods
	The JEA releases a public statement on the need to explain the relationship between epidemiology research and personal information to the public.
Apr. 2000	The Study Group on Development of Ethics Guidelines for Informed Consent in Epidemiologic Research issues the Guidelines on Informed Consent in Eepidemiological Studies, ver. 1.0.
	The Project Team of ethical ramifications and personal information protection in research and programs using epidemiologic methods is set up as a research project sponsored by MHW.
Jun. 2000	The Fundamental Principles of Research on the Human Genome is issued by the Council for Science and Technology, Bioethics Committee.
Oct. 2000	The Japanese government's Personal Information Protection Legislation Expert Committee (chaired by Itsuo Sonobe, former Supreme Court judge) announces an outline of the proposed Personal Information Protection Bill.
	The 5th revision of the Declaration of Helsinki (Edinburgh).
Mar. 2001	The Science Council of Japan the 7th Division (Medicine, Dentistry and Pharmaceutical Science) announces 'The Modality of Legislation Concerning the Protection of Personal Information in Medical Research'.
	The Association of Japanese Medical Colleges establishes the Subcommittee on Research Ethics.
	The Ethical Guidelines for Analytical Research on Human Genome/ Genes is announced as a result of continuous joint discussions by the Japanese Ministry of Education, Culture, Sports, Science and

Table A.1: continued

	Technology (MEXT), the Japanese Ministry of Health, Labour and Welfare (MHLW) and the Japanese Ministry of Economy, Trade and Industry (METI).
Apr. 2001	The Project Team of ethical ramifications and personal information protection in research and programs using epidemiologic methods announces the Guidelines on Bioethics and Personal Information Protection Issues in Epidemiological and Other Studies (draft) (the Maruyama Team Guidelines).
	MEXT, the MHLW and METI issue the Ethical Guidelines for Analytical Research on Human Genome/Genes.
	A Personal Information Protection Act fails during the regular session of the Diet. The proposed enforcement in April 2002 is put off.
May 2001	The Health Sciences Council Committee on Science and Technology sets up the *ad hoc* Committee on the Implementation of Research Using Epidemiologic Methods.
Aug. 2001	The Association of Japanese Medical Colleges Subcommittee on Research Ethics announces the Draft Guidelines on Epidemiological Research.
	The MEXT creates a Subcommittee on Research Using Epidemiologic Methods and drafts ethics guidelines for epidemiological research. This sub-committee belongs to the Bioethics and Safety Panel under the jurisdiction of the Council for Science and Technology Establishment of the IMJC for drafting a set of ethics guidelines.
Sep. 2001	MEXT announces the Guidelines for Derivation and Utilization of Human Embryonic Stem Cells.
Jan. 2002	The JEA announces an ethical proclamation for the conducting of epidemiological research.
Jun. 2002	The IMJC publishes the Ethical Guidelines for Epidemiological Research.
Oct. 2002	JEA announces the Ethical Guidelines for the Conduct of Ethical Studies and the JEA Terms and Conditions for the Establishment of Ethical Review Boards.
2002	CIOMS revises the International Ethical Guidelines for Biomedical Research Involving Human Subjects.
Oct.–Dec. 2002	The Bill for the Protection of Personal Information is abandoned during the 155th session of the Diet.
May 2003	The Act for the Protection of Personal Information is passed (after modification).
Jul. 2003	MHLW announces the Ethical Guidelines for Clinical Research.
Dec. 2004	The Two Ministry Joint Committee revises the Ethical Guidelines for Epidemiological Research (enforced in April 2005).
Jan. 2005	MHLW revises the Ethical Guidelines for Clinical Research (enforced in April 2005).
Apr. 2005	The Act for the Protection of Personal Information is enforced in full scale.

Index

Act for the Prevention of Misuse of Personal Data in Data Processing 244
Act on the Protection of Personal Information 250, 252
Advanced Information and Telecommunications Society Promotion Headquarters 243, 260
Agenda for Research on Women's Health for the 21st Century 145, 162
AGES project 190, 197
Aichi Gerontological Evaluation Study 136, 187
AIDS 85–7, 89, 129, 133, 140–1, 174, 180
Alameda County Study 169, 180, 205
alcohol 17, 31, 98–9, 122, 132, 136, 169, 177, 186, 189–90, 224, 236–7
alpha index 31–2
analytical epidemiology 253–4
Ancient Greek era 3
anomie 4
assets 22, 28, 62, 149
Association of Japanese Medical Colleges 247, 258, 261–2
attainment levels 123, 126

Basic Plan for Gender Equality 159
behavioural and cultural explanation 31, 35

Berkman, Lisa F. 1, 21, 23, 180, 200, 204–5, 238
bias 3, 31, 54, 165, 186, 243, 255
Bioethics and Biosafety Commission of the Council for Science and Technology 247
biological sex 144–51, 159–60
Black Report 30, 32, 35–6, 38
blood pressure 7, 10, 16–17, 65, 91, 99, 109, 114, 176, 216–21, 240, 252, 261
blue-collar workers 8, 91, 95–103, 108
Bond, Michael H. 167, 169–71, 173, 180
Bourdieu, Pierre 195
Britain 4, 9, 22, 30, 36, 41, 63, 70–1, 74, 170, 190
British Medical Journal 22–3, 38, 55, 62–5, 88–9, 111–13, 162–3, 239
bubble economy 40, 59

Canadian Ministry of Health 137
cancer 3, 70–1, 73, 92, 127–8, 130, 140–41, 171, 174, 177, 180, 186, 189, 205, 241, 243–4, 249, 251, 256, 259–61
 breast 127, 140, 171, 189
 cervical 70–1, 73, 140–1, 171
 epidemiology 3
cardiovascular epidemiology 3
Center for Epidemiologic Studies Depression Scale 105

cervical cancer screening 70–1, 127, 130
Chadwick, Edwin 4, 30, 36
Chernobyl 244
Chicago 67–9
child abuse 254
childbirth 148, 178
childrearing 148–9, 178, 186
China 27, 29, 170
chromosomes 148
chronic diseases 8, 127, 166
circulatory diseases 171, 176
cirrhosis 171, 173, 186
cognitive behavioral therapy 159
Coleman, James S. 194–5
Committee for Advanced Medical Technology Assessment of the Health Sciences Council 245
Committee on the Implementation of Research Using Epidemiologic Methods 247, 262
Committee on Understanding the Biology of Sex and Gender 145
Communicating with Seniors: Advice, Techniques and Tips 137
compositional effect 214
Comprehensive Survey of Living Conditions of the People on Health and Welfare 45, 51, 56, 59, 64, 236, 252
concavity effects 47–8
conception 2, 161
confounding factors 3, 59, 97, 127, 165
conjugal relations 184, 187

contextual effects 200, 215–16
conventional epidemiology 1, 7, 35, 240
Convention on the Elimination of All Forms of Discrimination against Women (CEDAW) 148, 159–60
conventional analysis models 217, 220
coronary heart disease 23, 90, 111–14, 176, 180
Council for International Organizations of Medical Sciences (CIOMS) 241–2, 246, 256, 259–60, 262
Guidelines 241–2, 246
cultural area 164–5, 168, 171, 174
cultural comparisons 170

Declaration of Helsinki 251, 259, 261
dementia 254
democracy 27, 205
Denmark 37, 113
DES (diethyl stilbestrol) 244
determinants of health 11, 20, 22–3, 38, 119, 122, 139, 182–3, 204, 211
Development Assistance Committee 29
diabetes 14, 125, 127–8, 131, 133, 135, 139–40, 211
diet 167, 175–7, 180, 189, 236, 237, 244, 262
diethyl stilbestrol *See* DES
discrimination 1, 2, 14, 16, 19, 23, 147–51, 159, 161–2
divorce 14, 184, 186–8, 237
Doi, Yuriko 144 152–5, 157–8, 16

domestic violence 254
drugs 76–81, 86, 122, 127, 129, 132–4, 179
Durkheim, David 196
Durkheim, Emile 4

ecologic fallacy *See* ecological fallacy
ecological 22, 42, 46, 54, 61–3, 199, 211, 213–14, 238, 252
 fallacy 46, 212
 studies 46, 62, 252
economic stability 189
education 4, 8, 12, 14, 16–18, 20, 31, 33, 35–6, 50, 60–2, 78, 90, 105–6, 117, 119–43, 164, 174–5, 183, 192, 195, 200, 204, 212–13, 223–5, 228, 230, 232–5, 238, 240–1, 253–6, 259, 261
elderly abuse 197, 199
emergency care 127, 132, 134
empirical studies 42, 95, 112, 193, 203
employment 1, 16, 20, 36, 46, 78, 94, 108, 110, 114, 124, 149, 160–1, 182, 186, 195, 237
England 32, 89, 90, 92, 111, 179, 180, 257
Ethical Guidelines for Analytical Research on Human Genome/Genes 247–8, 262
Ethical Guidelines for Clinical Studies 251
Ethical Guidelines for Epidemiological Research 240, 248–9, 256, 258–9, 262
Ethical Guidelines for the Conduct of Epidemiological Research 250
ethical review boards 249, 262
ethnicity 19–20, 36, 132, 141, 165, 167, 179
etiologic epidemiology 245
EU (European Union) 36, 139, 242, 244, 260
evidence-based medicine 260
excessive daytime sleepiness 156, 159, 163
exercise 61, 91, 136, 167, 183, 190, 200, 254

fallacies 46, 211–12, 238
 atomistic 212
 ecological/ecologic 46, 211–12
 psychologistic 212
 sociologistic 212
family 6–7, 15, 18, 33, 50, 61, 83, 139, 141–2, 157, 159, 161, 167, 169, 174, 182–4, 186, 189, 204
Finland 22, 190–1, 225
France 4, 41

gender 3, 16, 19, 31–2, 36, 42, 45, 50–2, 56, 60, 78, 80, 85, 96–7, 99–101, 103–6, 125, 127–8, 132, 144–151, 153, 155–63, 167–8, 178, 181, 218
Gender and Health (WHO report) 145, 162
genetics 2, 161
genotypes 237
geographic barriers 66–7
Geriatric Depression Scale 129, 187
Germany 4, 29, 170, 244, 259
Gestalt psychology 166

Gini index 18, 42–6, 48–52, 54–60, 74–5
GNP 13, 27, 29, 40, 170–3
Good Clinical Practice (GCP) 251
Gordis, Leon 244, 257, 259
Government Information and Individual Rights Subcommittee 244
Gravelle, Hugh 47–8, 63
Guidelines for Personal Information Protection and Bioethical Issues in Epidemiologic Research 247

Hamburg 244
Hanifan, Lydia Judson 195
Hashimoto, Hideki 21, 40, 64, 113, 239
hazardous activities 148, 160
hazardous environments 91
Health and Medical Service Law for the Aged 95
health care access 66–89, 194
health literacy assessment 134–5, 138
health risk avoidance 126–7, 132
Healthy People 2010 119, 137, 139
heart disease 8, 16, 23, 43, 90, 111–14, 170–3, 176, 180, 205, 211, 238
Helsinki 224, 226, 251, 259, 261
HIV 85–9, 125, 127, 129, 133, 139, 140–1, 143, 177, 241
anti-HIV combination therapy 85–7
HLM6 (software) 224

HMU (hypnotic medication use) 152, 154–5, 163
Hofstede, Geert 167, 170, 180
Honolulu 176
horizontal equity 88
household types 184
housework 149
hypertension 96, 99–100, 108–9, 113, 127–8, 139, 156, 171, 205, 211, 257
hypnotic medication 151–2, 154–5, 157–9, 163

IBM employees 167
immigrants 17, 20, 123, 138, 165, 174–6
income
  absolute 41, 46–8, 59
  relative 40–1, 48, 58–9, 194, 197
index of competence 136
India 27, 29, 170
individual-level social relationships 183
Industrial Revolution 4, 8, 90
infant deaths 31, 32, 33, 38
infectious diseases 3–4, 6, 10, 14–15, 32, 177–8
information technology (IT) 137–8, 178, 261
in-patient care 79, 81, 84, 127, 133
insomnia 151–3, 156, 163
Institute of Medicine (IOM), USA 145
insurance 50–1, 76, 78–9, 84–7, 89, 108, 123, 125–8, 132–3, 187, 207, 254
Inter-Ministry Joint Committee (IMJC) 247–8, 262

International Agency for Research on Cancer (IARC) 244
International Year of Older Persons 137
internet 137, 177
intraclass correlation 216, 237
inverse care law 70, 88
ischemic heart disease 8, 43, 113, 171–2, 205, 211, 238
Israel 59, 65
Italy 41, 76, 195, 202
Iwata, Noboru 164

Japan Collaborative Cohort Study for the Evaluation of Cancer Risk (JACC study) 241, 256, 260
Japan Epidemiological Association (JEA) 22, 114, 241–2, 245–6, 250, 257, 260–2
  Sub-committee of Ethical Issues 241
Japan International Cooperation Agency (JICA) 30
Japan Society for Occupational Health 246, 257
Japanese Diet (Japanese Parliament) 250
Japanese Ministry of Education, Culture, Sports, Science and Technology (MESC, MEXT) 240, 246–50, 256, 261–2
Japanese Ministry of Health, Labour and Welfare (MHLW, MHW) 240, 242–4, 247–8, 250, 256–7, 260–2
Japanese National Health Insurance 108
Japanese Pharmaceutical Affairs Law 251
Japanese Society of Public Health 246
Jichi Medical School Cohort Study 95, 113

Kawachi, I. 1, 15, 21–3, 47–9, 51, 53, 57, 58, 60, 62–5, 163, 197, 200, 203–6, 238
Kawakami, Norito 1, 21, 103, 108, 112–14
Kenya 27, 29
Kishiwada City 32–3
Kobayashi, Yasuki 27, 38, 40, 75, 89, 113–14
Kondō Katsunori 182

language 16, 19, 20, 138, 145, 164–5, 167–8, 175–6, 179
lifestyle 3, 6, 8, 16, 19, 31, 35–6, 60–1, 65, 119, 121–2, 127, 132, 137, 139, 153, 164–7, 169, 174–8, 183, 189, 211, 222, 237–8, 240, 253
living environment 35–6
London 5, 8, 22, 88–9, 112, 139–40, 179–80, 224, 238
Lorenz curve 74–5

macro-level culture 169
macro-level data 42
macro-social factors 2, 161
marital status 17, 50–2, 56, 60, 124, 129, 157, 184, 186, 188, 237

marriage 178, 182–90, 204
Maruyama, Eiji 246–7, 256, 258, 262
Maruyama, Hiroshi 31–3, 38
Maruyama Team 246–7, 262
Massachusetts 37–8, 179
materialist/structural explanation 31, 35
mediation mechanism 95, 95
Medicare 123–5, 129–31, 133–4, 139–41
mental health 3–4, 22, 141, 149–50, 175, 180, 187, 192, 201
meso-level culture 168, 174, 176
micro-level culture 176, 177
migrant communities 174, 178
Millennium Development Goals 29, 38
Ministry of Health and Social Security (UK) 30
MLwiN software 50–1, 224, 238
Modality of Legislation Concerning the Protection of Personal Information in Medical Research 246, 261
MONICA study 96
mortality rate 5, 13, 15–16, 30–2, 37, 41–7, 59, 71, 73, 90–1, 196–7, 227, 232, 234–5, 237
multilevel analysis 11, 36, 38, 46, 48, 50–3, 63–4, 166, 169, 176, 211–39
multilevel modelling 49, 221, 238
Multilevel Models Project of the Institute of Education 224

multinational companies 178
mutual distrust 196
mutual support 171, 196, 201–2

Nakayama, Takeo 22, 240, 256–8
National Adult Literacy Survey (NALS) 121, 123, 126, 139
national census 45, 50, 52, 67, 152, 224, 252
National Health Service (NHS), UK 70, 89
National Institute of Health (NIH), USA 145, 162
National Nutrition Survey 252
neighbourhood 2, 38, 65, 161, 239
neo-materialism 60
neoplasms 171–2
Netherlands 76–7, 170, 259
Ni-Hon-San Study 17, 176
Nishi, Nobuo 22, 211, 238
nursing care 149, 157–8, 185, 205, 207, 254
nutritional counselling 35

obesity 91, 190, 254
occupational class 15–16, 31–2, 36, 90–115, 237–8
OECD 29, 243–4, 259
  8 principles 243–4
old age 2, 123–6, 137, 161
Osaka 32, 44
out-patient care 79, 81, 84

Personal Information Protection Bill 246, 249–50, 261
Personal Information Protection Investigative Subcommittee 243, 260

Personal Information Protection Legislation Expert Committee 246, 261
Petty, William 27
pharmacotherapy 159
phototherapy 159
physical exercise 190, 200
physicians 27, 66–71, 74, 84, 99, 122–32, 143, 260
Pittsburgh Sleep Quality Index (PSQI), 151, 156
plague 27
plasma fibrinogen 91, 96–98, 109, 113–14, 176
policy epidemiology 245
politics 62, 149, 164, 196, 227
pollution effects 47–8
poverty 1, 4, 13–14, 18, 27–40, 52, 64, 124
  absolute 29, 30, 35–6
  anti-poverty programs 27
  relative 28
prescriptions 76–7, 80, 89, 134, 142
preventive care 70, 85, 127, 132
price sensitivity 76–8
principle of consent 243–4
privacy 240, 243–5, 248, 252–4, 257, 259, 261
PROC MIXED (software) 224
PROC NLMIXED (software) 224
professional workers 90
Project Team for the Study of Ethical Ramifications and Personal Data Protection in Research and Programs Using Epidemiologic Methods 246
psychosocial factors 111–14

psychosocial job stress 91, 94–5, 106
psychosocial stress 179, 201
public statistics 251–2
Putnam, Robert 194–5, 201–2, 205–6

race 16, 19–20, 36, 50–2, 64, 124–8, 140, 165, 167, 169, 179, 190
RAND Health Insurance Experiment 78–9, 84–5, 89
Rapid Estimate of Adult Literacy in Medicine (REALM) 124–5, 128–30, 134–8, 143
reciprocal relationships 1
reciprocity 113, 195, 198, 200
reproduction 62, 142
risk ratios 227–33
rural areas 67, 69–70
Russia 27, 40, 62

San Francisco 125, 131, 176, 205
sanitary conditions 4, 8
SAS macro GLIMMIX (software) 50, 224, 227
Saving Lives: Our Healthier Nation 119, 139
schools 135, 167–8, 213, 223, 246
Science Council of Japan 246, 257, 261
self-care 126, 127, 132, 139
semi-skilled workers 90
Seventh-day Adventists 176, 180
single causal factor theories 4
skilled workers 90, 100–3
smoking 6, 8, 11, 16–17, 31, 35, 50, 60, 91, 98–9, 127,

129, 132, 136, 140, 167, 169, 183, 186, 189–90, 211, 236–7, 254
anti-smoking 35
social capital 15, 19, 23, 35–6, 58, 61, 65, 136, 168, 182–3, 194–207
social classes 4–8, 12–13, 15, 17–18, 20–1, 32, 36, 60, 92, 111, 113, 168–9, 190, 195, 225, 229–35
social determinants of health 11, 20, 22–3, 38, 119, 139, 204
social epidemiological paradigm 150–1, 160
social integration 23, 167–71, 195–6
social networks 15, 18, 23, 36, 167, 169, 180–4, 189–91, 194, 204–5
social norms 4, 122, 250
social order 4
social relationships 12, 15, 18–19, 62, 182–207
Social Security Scheme (SSS) 86
social selection explanation 31
social sex 144, 146–50, 158–60
social structure 1, 3–4, 6–12, 17, 20–1, 120–7, 164, 195
social support 7, 15, 18–20, 23, 65, 130–1, 140, 171, 182–5, 189–94, 204–5
social support-networks 184–5, 189, 192
socioeconomic status 1, 10, 17, 60, 62–3, 90, 109, 112, 114, 119, 127–8, 132, 142, 186, 190, 192, 204, 211, 237, 239

socio-medical paradigm 150, 160
socio-occupational class 31–2, 36
Soviet Union 40, 244
Spasoff, Robert 245, 257
Special Cancer Research Organization 241
spouses 19, 158, 159, 184, 187, 189
Springfield 68–9
standardized mortality ratios 113
Study on Assessment of Epidemiologic Research in Terms of Contributions to Health Policy 245, 257, 261
Study on the Development of Ethics Guidelines for Informed Consent in Epidemiologic Research 242, 257
Subcommittee on Studies Using Epidemiological Methods 247
subcultures 168, 179
Sugimori, Hiroki 119
Sweden 9, 76, 170, 190–1, 259

Taiwan 59, 65, 170
Tamakoshi, Akiko 242
tax system 4
Test of Functional Health Literacy in Adults (TOFHLA) 123–5, 128–31, 134–5, 142
Thailand 85–6, 89, 170
time-series analysis 45–6, 58–9, 65
Titanic 1, 21
tobacco 122, 140, 177

Tokyo Metropolitan Institute of Gerontology 136
Townsend Deprivation Index 71
Toyokawa, Satoshi 66
Tsutsumi, Akizumi 90, 97–8, 103, 112–15
Tudor Hart, Julian 70
typhus 4

uncertainty avoidance 167, 178
UNESCO 121, 164, 166, 179
United Nations 29, 148, 159
universal coverage scheme 86
unskilled workers 90
urban areas 69, 70, 153
US National Academies' Institute of Medicine *See* Institute of Medicine
US National Institute of Health *See* National Institute of Health

value dimensions 167, 170–2
variables
  aggregate 213, 223
  environmental 214
  global 214, 222
  individual-level 36, 55–6, 212–13, 220–36
  population-level 36
  regional-level 53
vertical equity 88
Villermé, Louis-René 4
Virchow, Rudolph 4, 22, 27

wages 149
Wales 32, 90, 92, 111
white-collar workers 18, 91, 97–103, 105, 108–9, 163
Whitehall II Study 22, 107, 111–14

Wide Range Achievement Test (WRAT) 135–6
Wilkinson, Richard 22,–3, 38, 40–2, 62, 65, 139, 204, 206
Woolcock, Michael 201
Work, Lipids and Fibrinogen (WOLF) Study 107–9
World Bank 13, 29, 30, 33–4, 38, 194, 201, 206
World Development Report 1993 33, 36, 38
World Health Organization (WHO) 20, 23, 29, 38, 120–1, 145–6, 150, 162–3, 206
World War II 3, 59, 147